MW00886403

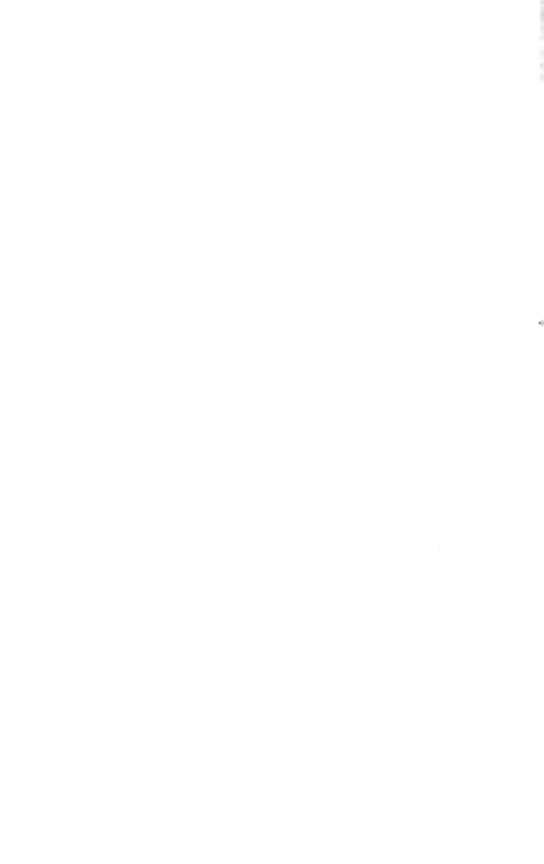

How to Make Herbal Incense

Step-by-Step Blueprint on How to Make Your Own Herbal Incense

(Including Over 50 Recipes to Get Started)

Introduction

Have you tried different types of store-bought incense, but they've all caused you discomfort, such as choking, headaches, or allergies that diminish the perceived benefits?

Are you interested in creating your herbal incense with full control over its ingredients, allowing for a natural and fulfilling way to create a calming atmosphere in your home?

Would you like a comprehensive guide that reveals all the necessary information to make your herbal incense, enabling you to enjoy its numerous benefits and eliminate the need to purchase traditional incense in the future?

If you have answered YES, this book provides the blueprint for crafting your own herbal incense to transform your home into a sanctuary without feeling like you are trying too hard!

Studies published in the Natural Library of Medicine, such as one published by professors Ta Ching Lin, Guka Krishnaswamy, and David S Chi[1] in 2008, give the dirty secret behind the state of most incense today.

---

[1] **https://www.ncbi.nlm.nih.gov/pmc/articles/PMC2377255/**

Averagely, incense produces more particles in the air than other smoke-producing substances, such as cigarettes (incense produces 45 mg/g while cigarettes produce 10 mg/g). This quantity of smoke is too much whether you are using herbal or standard incense, don't you agree?

It does not stop here.

Incense does not only produce gases such as CO, SO_2, NO_2, and CO_2; it emits more volatile compounds such as polycyclic aromatic hydrocarbons, xylenes, toluene, and benzene, which all lead to air pollution, high levels of cord blood IgE, allergic contact dermatitis, and respiratory system dysfunction among others.

Look at the image below;

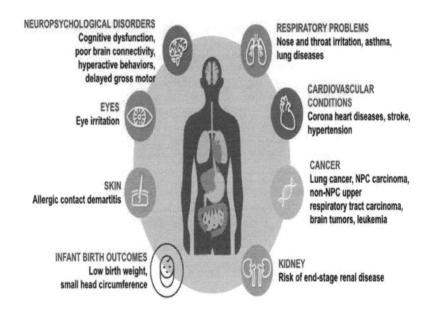

NEUROPSYCHOLOGICAL DISORDERS
Cognitive dysfunction, poor brain connectivity, hyperactive behaviors, delayed gross motor

RESPIRATORY PROBLEMS
Nose and throat irritation, asthma, lung diseases

CARDIOVASCULAR CONDITIONS
Corona heart diseases, stroke, hypertension

EYES
Eye irritation

CANCER
Lung cancer, NPC carcinoma, non-NPC upper respiratory tract carcinoma, brain tumors, leukemia

SKIN
Allergic contact demartitis

INFANT BIRTH OUTCOMES
Low birth weight, small head circumference

KIDNEY
Risk of end-stage renal disease

Fig: Effects of poorly made incense

Now since there is no 'safe smoke' when it comes to making incense, one of the questions I asked myself was...

What can I do to get the full benefits of herbal incense without endangering myself with the smoke it produces?

This question is the driving force of this book;

The good news is there is a way to make incense such that when you ignite it, the amount of smoke produced comes off lighter than usual!

But to do this, I am sure you have questions such as...

What herbs and resins should I use to make incense?

Should I use fresh or dried herbs to make my incense?

What are the main ingredients of herbal incense?

What are the right mixing measurements that I should use?

How do I blend scents to create a unique fragrance?

How can I use incense to unlock its full range of benefits?

How will I know if my incense is of great quality?

If these are the questions you have, then you are reading the right book because it will answer them and more in simple language!

In this book, you will learn:

- The basics, including the types and varieties of incense and different incense scents

- Different types of herbs used to make incense

- List of other ingredients and the right measurements required to make herbal incense

- The properties of different herbs and resins and how to choose the right ones

- How to make different types of incense, including cones and sticks

- Safety precautions to consider before making herbal incense

- How to blend scents to create unique fragrances

- How to use incense for meditation and spiritual practices

- Tips for storing and burning incense safely

- Recipe development, including how to create your recipes as a pro, key fundamentals to consider before making them, and how to create stunning recipe templates

- Herbal incense recipes to help you get started

...and much more!

So, whether you want to create a relaxing atmosphere in your home or enhance your spiritual practice without worrying about your respiratory system or illnesses that come with poorly-created incense, this beginner's guide to making herbal incense is the perfect place to start your journey to making a natural, safe, and easy way to create beautiful scents for your home!

Without much further ado, let'ss get right into it!

PS: I'd like your feedback. If you are happy with this book, please leave a review on Amazon.

Please leave a review for this book on Amazon by visiting the page below:

https://amzn.to/2VMR5qr

Table of Contents

Section 1: The Building Blocks of Incense

Every incense is made from the following main components;

- Scent

- Base

- Liquid

- Color

- Bonding Agent

Let us discuss each of them.

Chapter 1: The Scent

The scent is the aroma of the incense – the part that gives the incense its characteristic fragrance. As you would guess, there are so many things that can be used to bring out the distinctive aroma of incense, some of which include:

- Essential oils

- Herbs

- Spices

- Resins

- Artificial fragrances

It is this part of incense that gives it the sought-after benefits such as:

- Providing a calming effect while stimulating the senses

- Purifying the air

- Improving the mood

- Cleansing the air

- Quieting the mind

- Stimulating creativity

- Enhancing concentration

- Promoting good quality sleep

- Providing the benefits of aromatherapy

...among others.

These benefits can only be brought about by the substances used in making the incense. Suppose you use artificial substances that may have harmful effects as opposed to therapeutic effects. In that case, you cannot expect to reap the benefits of your incense.

More precisely, most store-bought incense is made using petroleum-based chemical compounds such as phthalates, styrene, and benzophenone that have been linked to different harmful effects on the body like cancers, kidney diseases, asthma, liver tumor, mammary gland tumors, skin, throat and eye irritations[2] and many others.[3]

This is why it is crucial to gravitate towards using natural sources of the scent to avoid exposing yourself to potentially harmful substances while also ensuring you get the full range of benefits that come with using ingredients with therapeutic benefits.

Our focus for this book will be pure essential oils, natural herbs, resins, and spices as sources of scents.

---

[2] https://www.ncbi.nlm.nih.gov/pmc/articles/PMC2377255/
[3] https://www.ncbi.nlm.nih.gov/pmc/articles/PMC8548258/

Natural Herbs

Herbs have a characteristic natural scent that can make your incense quite therapeutic if incorporated well.

Some of the most popular herbs in making incense include the following:

- Thyme

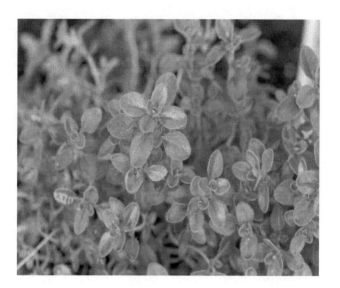

- Sage

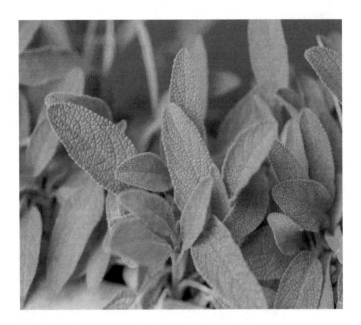

- Rosemary

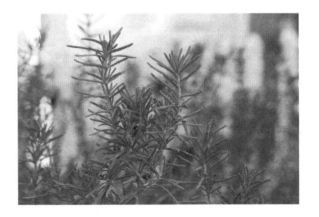

- Peppermint

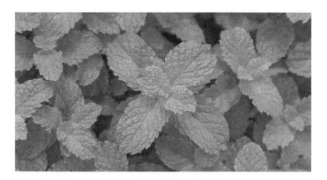

- Marjoram

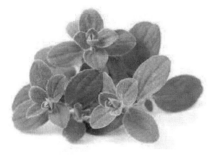

- Lavender

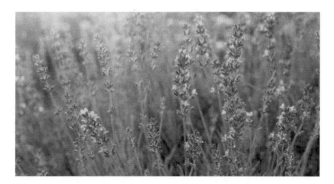

- Hyssop

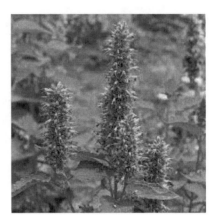

- Dill

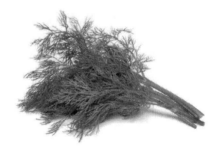

- Catnip

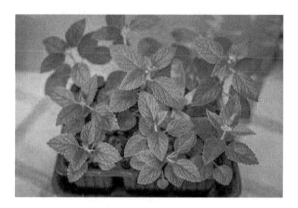

- Basil

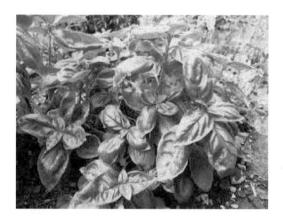

And the good thing with herbs is that they are easy to extract - if you have herbs in your garden and the growing season is upon you, harvest them by cutting the sprigs right above the chives, leaf clusters, barks, or stems (remember this depends on what part of the herb is required).

You can use the following basic steps to create incense from all or most of these parts. However, this is just to give you an idea of what to expect when creating different recipe:

- First, gather all the dried herbs that you need.

- Crush these dried herbs into powder.

- Add makko powder (this is a binding agent – we will discuss this later in subsequent sections) into the ground mixture, then mix well.

- Add some distilled water to the mixture, then mold the cones.

- Allow the dough to dry, then shape them.

- Finally, light the incense, and enjoy!

You can also make incense using fresh herbs.

(The steps below involve making incense with fresh herbs and flowers):

- Harvest, prepare, then bundle the herbs. The preparation involves cutting the stems and then removing the flowers.

- Secure the bundled herbs and flowers.

- Hang these bundles upside down to dry for at least 14 days.

- Finally, place the dry bundles on an incense burner or any other heat-proof plate, then light it.

Essential Oils

Essential oils are oils specially extracted from plants through processes such as:

- Steam distillation

- Solvent extraction

- CO2 extraction

- Cold-press extraction or expression

- Water distillation

- Enfleurage

- Maceration

These processes are quite complex, and outside the scope of this book, so we will not go into detail on them. What you should ensure is that you get authentic essential oils obtained using any of these methods to make the incense we will be making throughout the book.

Some of the most common oils used in making incense include the following:

- Ylang ylang complete

- Vanilla

- Sweet orange

- Spruce

- Spearmint

- Sandalwood

- Rosemary

- Rose geranium

- Rose damascene

- Rosalina patchouli

- Palo santo

- Palmarosa

- Opopanax

- Myrrh

- Lemongrass

- Lavandin super

- Juniper berry

- Hemlock

- Grapefruit

- Ginger, fresh

- Frankincense

- Clary sage

- Chocolate peppermint

- Cedarwood

- Bergamot

Here are some steps to follow when using essential oils as scents for your incense:

- First, measure the essential oils you need. For sticks, each incense stick needs 20 drops of oil.

- Place unscented incense sticks on a dish or any container covered with foil paper.

- Pour the oil into the dish and ensure the sticks fully suck in the essential oils.

- Allow the incense sticks to dry off, then light them when ready.

Resins

Incense resins are natural substances that are harvested from gum trees through a process known as tapping. Before incense sticks were used, resin incense was the original incense, and if you use it, as we will in subsequent chapters, you will agree that it gives off a richer and deeper fragrance!

So, as you will see later on, using resins to produce scent is easy.

All you need is to place salt or sand inside an incense burner (this boosts heat absorption). Then, place a charcoal tablet on the burner and finally light it.

There are different types of resins that you can use in your incense. Some of these include:

- Seven chakra resin

- Frankincense and myrrh resin

- Sweet frankincense resin

- Dragon's Blood resin

- Benzoin of Sumatra resin

- Mayan copal resin

- Frankincense and sandalwood blend resin

- Kashmir resin

- Black Ethiopian resin

- Myrrh select resin

Spices

As we mentioned earlier, spices also chip into the aroma of the incense. There are two main categories of spices:

- Fresh spices – these spices are better used as top notes (we will learn all about notes later in this chapter).

The following are examples of fresh spices that work perfectly with incense:

- o Juniper berries

- o Ginger

- o Timut pepper

- o Pink pepper

- o Coriander

- o Cardamom

- Hot spices – these spices are better used as base/leg notes.

The following are the most common examples used as hot/warm spices:

- o Pepper berries

- o Saffron

- o Peppers

- o Cinnamon wood

- o Mace and nutmeg

With all these different varieties of aromas to choose from, using more than one may cause some confusion. To help with this, you need to know more about how these fragrances work so that when blending them, you do it without making avoidable mistakes. Let us learn this next.

Incense Scent Notes

As you learn how to make incense, you need to understand the concept of notes:

When you light your herbal incense, the first smell that reaches your nose is **"the head."** This is the lightest scent and will fade fastest (between 0 and 15 minutes after lighting the incense).

After it fades off, the incense's scent will still linger in the air, but it will be combined with the next scent known as **'the heart.'** The 'heart' is deeper and stronger and lasts for around 20 to 60 minutes. It is at this stage that the herb's real scent becomes clearer.

After 60 minutes or so, the last wave of scent takes over (we can title this final wave **the Legs**). The aroma is at its strongest here and, with some help (we will discuss this later in subsequent chapters), can linger in the air longer, even after the incense burns out.

This is an interesting process, right? Remember this process because it will help you choose the best scent to use when blending different scents (do not worry about this now. We will discuss more later).

Chapter 2: The Bases

As we mentioned earlier, every burned scent has three main notes: head, heart, and legs. These three notes are made from different natural materials such as wood, bamboo, sawdust, or charcoal (these materials burn slowly and evenly, which makes the fragrance burn longer).

To understand how these different bases work, let us group them into notes:

1. The Head

As we mentioned, the head is the first scent you will smell, lasting anywhere between 5 to 15 minutes. Many things can be used as bases, such as yuzu, sweet orange, sandalwood, Ravensara, pine, petitgrain, palmarosa, nutmeg, and rosewood, among others, but we will focus on herbs.

The following are some of the herbs that you can use as top bases:

- **Basil**

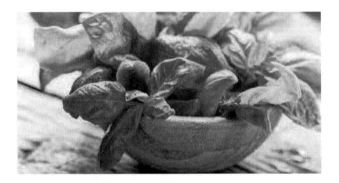

Basil provides some intense freshness which lasts for around 15 minutes minimum and 1 hour maximum (after this time, it evaporates fast).

- **Violet**

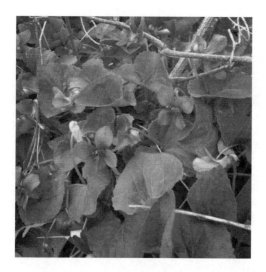

Some use this herb as a middle note because it lends a powerful and intense green note to scents which is reminiscent of cut grass, cucumber peels, and hay.

- **Tuberose**

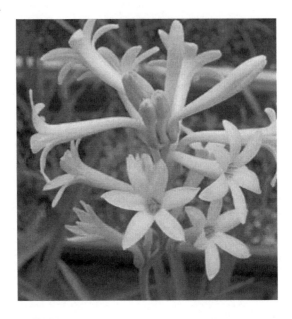

This herb has a narcotic odor and a strong, seductive ointment scent, making it perfect for use as a top note.

- **Thyme**

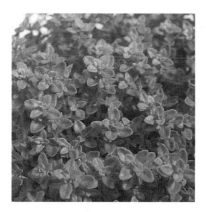

Thyme's scent closely resembles oregano's, but it is more resinous and, to some extent, takes the scent direction of rosemary. Kindly note that as much as thyme is used as a top note, using it primarily does not have the best scent, so use it with a combination of other scents for a better outcome.

- **Tea tree**

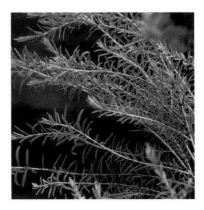

This herb is considered a head or a body type of scent note. It is used in both clusters because it is more concentrated as compared to other scents. So, this depends on you – if you need an herb that will last longer immediately, go for tea tree because it can linger in the air for up to two hours!

- **Tagetes**

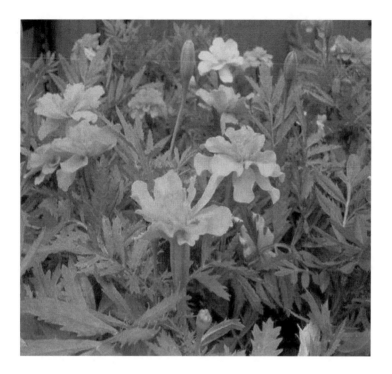

This herb produces a fresh herbaceous aroma that comes with some green apple and floral scents. It is perfect as a top note because it complements other fragrances, such as citrus and others from the wood and floral families.

- **Sweet marjoram**

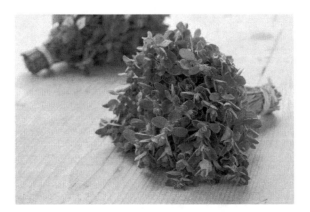

This herb is dual – meaning it can be used as a head and body note. It has a medium scent strength and is warm and spicy (you might also smell some nutmeg).

- **Roman Chamomile**

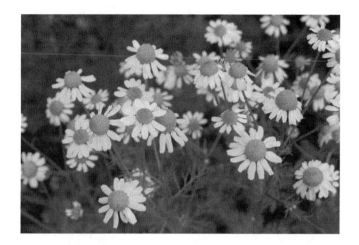

This herb is perfect as a top note because it perfectly links fruity, citrusy notes and floral scents and is pretty fleeting. However, if you use German varieties such as Matricaria chamomilla, I recommend using it as a top and middle note.

- **Mimosa**

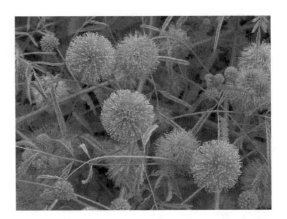

This is an enriching herb meaning it complements head and leg notes. It has a warm, powdery, and honey scent and supports jasmine, rose, and tuberose herbs well.

- **Melissa**

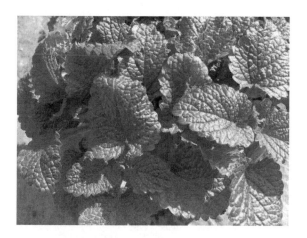

Melissa, or lemon balm, is a perfect top scent because it effortlessly blends with other scents. Specifically, it has a warm, lemony note with a unique herbaceous balsamic undertone.

- **Linden blossom**

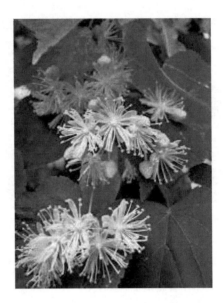

This herb is a good head note because it is not very strong. It fades fast and can also be used as a binding agent (we will discuss more about this later).

- **Lavandin**

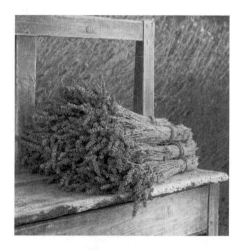

This herb is quite versatile because, as you will see, it is a potent modifier and blends well with many other raw herbs and their essential oils.

- **Ginger**

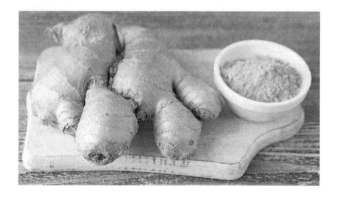

This herb is perfect for use as a top note due to its effervescence and freshness. However, kindly note that you will feel it until the incense is burnt through – yes, it is that strong, so do not be afraid to use it as a head, heart, or leg.

- **Galbanum**

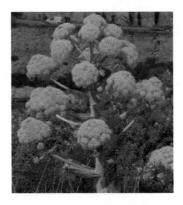

Galbanum is a head note that gives the incense a rich natural effect to other fragrances such as violet, iris, narcissus, gardenia, and hyacinth, among others. You can also burn hyacinth on its own, but only consider this if you fancy brash scents.

- **Coriander**

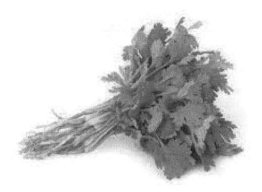

This is a men's choice note that primarily acts as a head note but can also be used as a middle note. Its strength is considered medium strong, sweet, and a little fruity, and if you let it age (I will show you how to do this later), it will enhance the fragrance to insane levels.

- **Cardamom**

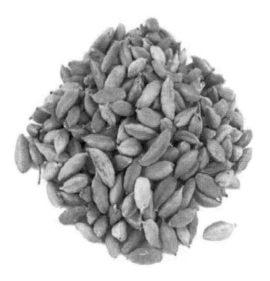

You can use this herb as a head or a heart note since its warm, spicy, and light sweet aroma adds depth, complexity, and uniqueness to the other notes, thus creating a scent that lingers for long.

2. The Heart

The heart notes consist of scents that last approximately 20 to 60 minutes. The herbs used here are more dominant, making them linger longer as compared to top notes.

The following are the most common herbs used as heart or middle notes:

- **Hyacinth**

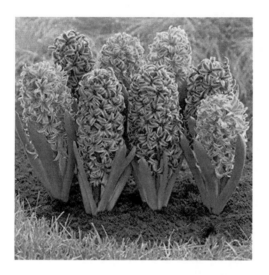

Hyacinth is a complex and powerful fragrance with a flowery and sweet undertone. You can use it either as a head or a heart note. However, we recommend using it as a heart note since it lasts more.

- **Geranium/cranesbill**

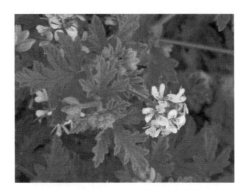

This herb base is considered one of the best heart bases known because it perfectly bonds the head and the leg. This means that it will give a boost to all the other bases you use, thus making it last longer and equally stronger.

- **Black pepper**

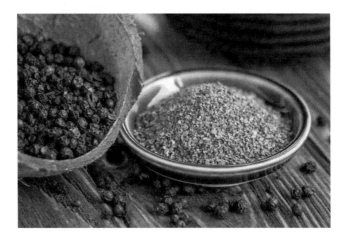

This herb is perfect for combining the top and leg notes because it perks up and adds spice and heat to the mixture. You also do not have to be cautious about using black pepper because it blends with floral, citrus, and spice notes!

- **Bay**

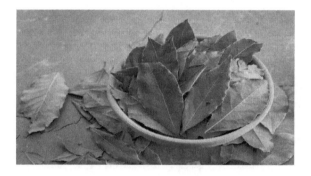

This herb leaf is spicy and powerful, making it a perfect choice for the heart notes. Kindly note that this herb works well with most masculine fragrances.

- **Yarrow**

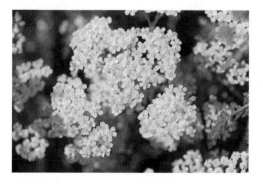

This herb has a sweet diffusive scent that is sweet, fresh, woody, and green-herbaceous. These unique properties make it perfect for blending with other plants in other notes, thus making it a middle note.

- **Violet**

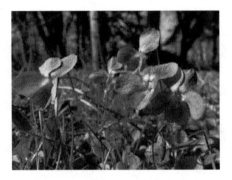

This herb has a singular scent of fresh cucumber and cuts grass. It is considered a heart note because it produces an elegance rarely achieved with any other note. This is why it blends well with hyacinth, lily of the valley, basil, cumin, sage, tuberose, and narcissus, among others.

- **Vetiver**

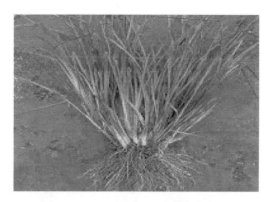

Vetiver produces a scent considered attractive, warm, dry, and earthy. The scent produced is grounding and sensuous in nature, blending well with all kinds of fragrances in other notes.

- **Tuberose**

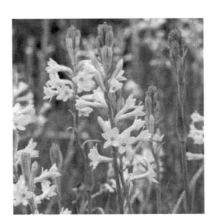

This herb has a floral, sweet honey scent. Since its overall scent is considered captivating, especially for feminine fragrances, you can use it as a heart note.

You can also use other plants and flowers like:

- **Ylang ylang**

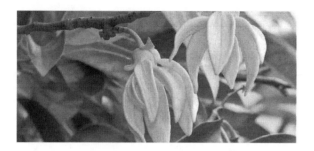

This shrub produces a gentle, delicious, floral scent that is somehow like jasmine. When first used, the scent is floral and sweet, but it becomes mild and more pleasant after a while.

Ylang-ylang is used as a heart base because it is low-priced and has a rich and complex scent that blends well with mimosa, tuberose, gardenia, bergamot, opoponax, amyl salicylate, and vetiver, among others.

- **Myrrh**

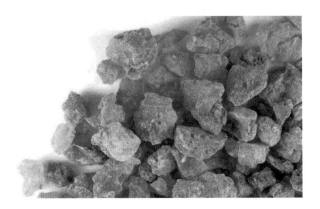

This sap-like substance, also known as a resin, has a rich, warm, spicy scent with a unique balsamic undertone. You can use it to strengthen the head notes because it has medium strength.

- **Jasmine**

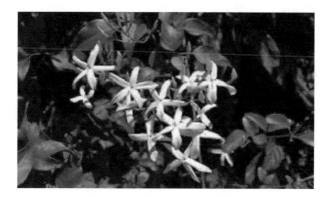

Jasmine has a sweet, rich, fruity, and sensual scent that can be perfectly used as a heart note. It will provide a strong initial impression and contribute to the strength of the entire fragrance.

- **Labdanum**

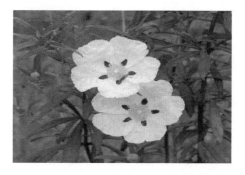

This herb has a strong, warm, sweet, musky, fruity, amber scent. Use this note to add some warmth and sweetness to a fragrance.

You can also use it as a leg note to provide longevity, depth, and structure. What to note is that it is long-lasting, evaporates slowly, and helps ground the fragrance.

The Leg

The herbs used in this note are the strongest and can last at least 6 hours. They have strong, heavy molecular structures and are less volatile than herbs used for top and middle notes.

The following are some of the common leg note herbs known today:

- **Oakmoss**

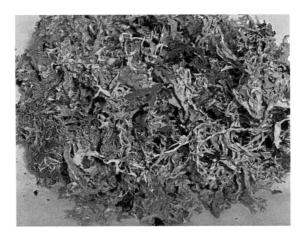

This herb is sometimes used as a head note, but we recommend using it as a leg note because it perfectly anchors volatile scents such as citrus scents. In addition, another reason for recommending using oakmoss as a base is it is so unique that it is blacklisted in some countries in its oil form for being an allergen (however, it is safe to use as a raw herb).

- **Valerian**

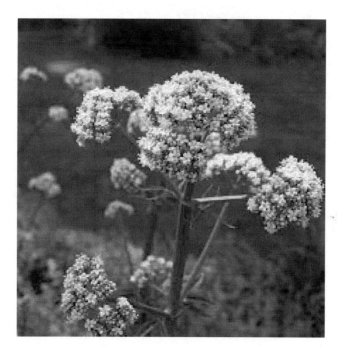

Valerian has a balsamic, musky green, grounding scent that works well if used as a base or leg note. You can blend it with yarrow spikenard, patchouli, lavender, and copaiba balsam, among others.

- **Balsam Peru**

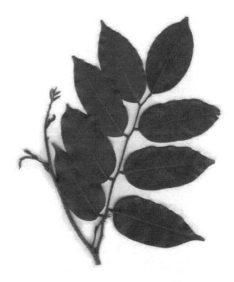

This herb has rich, sweet, smooth, caramel, and vanilla scents, making it a strong base fixative of these and any scents with most woods, the favorite being sandalwood.

You can also use other plants, such as:

- **Sandalwood**

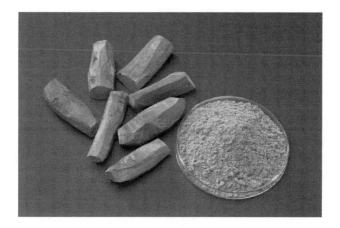

This tree produces a bright, fresh scent that acts as a fixative that complements and enhances other notes.

- **Bay**

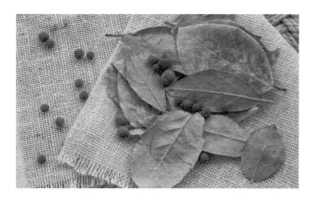

This herb produces a green, herbal note with a touch of thyme, cypress, laurel leaf, vetiver, cedarwood, and oregano.

- **Balsam**

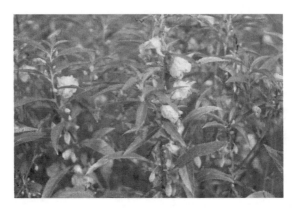

This herb produces a scent like vanilla but has a hint or two of cinnamon. Balsam will help alter the strength of any flowery notes you might be using to make your incense, thus making it long-lasting.

The following are not herbs but can be used as bases for your incense;

- **Cedarwood**

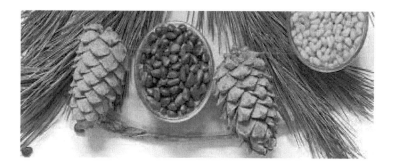

This is a tree that produces a fragrance that anchors the top and middle notes. Use it with floral and citrus notes because it lends some unique warmth, but you can also use it with musk and amber notes because it produces a clean green aroma with a vintage/retro vibe.

- **Benzoin**

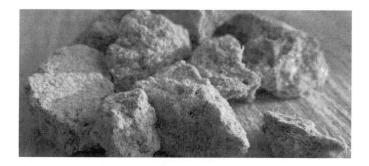

Benzoin is a resin from the bark of a tree. It has a sweet, warm scent that is used as a base, especially if you want to create a fragrance with a medium aroma and a touch of vanilla.

As we have seen in this section, there are many fragrances to choose from. What might pose a challenge is knowing how to blend them perfectly. To do this, you need to know how to use what is known as the fragrance wheel.

Let us discuss this next.

Chapter 3: The Fragrance Wheel

A fragrance wheel, which is also known as an aroma or perfume wheel, is simply a circular diagram that tells us more about how notes should be mixed or blended. Since 1979 when notable versions of fragrance wheels appeared, many versions have been produced.

However, the most common version used today is the 1992 brainchild of Michael Edwards[4], a renowned expert perfumer and taxonomist.

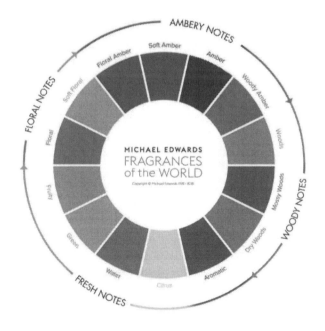

---

4   https://www.researchgate.net/figure/Michael-Edwards-perfume-fragrance-wheel_fig1_266510755

You might be wondering, how exactly does this wheel help? Well...

Normally, there are basic scents that are known to complement each other, but because you want to create incense that solely matches what you want and need, you might need to sample a few fragrances. This is where the wheel comes in – it will help guide you better.

This wheel is split into four main sections. They are:

- Floral

- Oriental or also known as amber

- Woody

- Fresh

These four sections have more sub-scents that are quite like each other, scents that share complement each other, and ones that share the same characteristics.

With this brief introduction in mind, let us go deeper and discuss more regarding the scent families that we have just listed:

The Fresh Family

This family consists of refreshing and vibrant scents. This means the plants involved should be bright, herbal, oceanic, and citrus-based. They can also be woody but be keen not to add too much of it because it will destroy the scent in totality.

If you will use luxurious scents such as sage, amber, lemon, coconut, coffee, lavender, rose, and vanilla, blend them with spicy scents such as juniper, ginger, timut, pink pepper, coriander, and cardamon, zesty scents such as lemons, grapefruit, and clementine, and aromatic scents such as sage, mint, and rosemary. This combination will give you a uniquely rich, fresh family scent that blows your mind!

The fresh family consists of the following sub-types:

- Aromatic fresh – this subtype consists of basil, lavender, rosemary, and other woody scents such as cedarwood, vetiver, patchouli, pine, and sandalwood.

- Citrus fresh – this subtype consists of bright scents that are blended with bergamot, citrus, mandarin, grapefruit, and lush orange.

- Water fresh – this subtype consists of aquatic and marine scents. This means using coastal or aquatic, citrus, and woody plants.

- Green fresh – this subtype includes herbal, fresh, and leafy scents such as basil, parsley, cilantro, mint, rosemary, thyme, chives, and sage.

- Fruity fresh – this subtype has scents that lie between floral and fresh scents of the fragrance wheel. So you can use scents such as apple, pear, and velvet, among others.

The Floral Family

The scents under this section have freshly cut flowers, and because they are many, classifying them depends on how intense you want them to be and what other scents you would like to add to them.

To make blending easier, the floral section is further divided into:

- **Floral flesh**

To attain that fresh scent, the scents you should blend here must be from herbs that have woody, spicy, smoky, and bright flowered scents. So, to get that fresh floral fragrance from your herbs, blend a herb or two from the following sections:

- o Woody herbs – these include tarragon, thyme, sweet bay, sage, lavender, and rosemary.

- o Spicy herbs – these include black cumin, bergamot, basil, bay leaf, asafoetida, anise, angelica, and allspice, among others.

- o Smoky herbs – these include sage, mint, uva-ursi, mugwort, coltsfoot, skullcap, and mullein, among others.

- o Flowering herbs – these include bee balm, lavender, Thai basil, dill, rosemary, Greek oregano, spearmint, and pineapple sage, among others.

- **Soft floral**

Soft floral fragrances consist of powdery scents such as amber, opoponax resin, heliotrope, musks, rose, vanilla, violet, sandalwood, patchouli, balsam, oakmoss, and iris/orris.

- **Floral amber**

This sub-section must have assorted sweet spices and floral orange blossom spices. This, therefore, means you can blend the following herbs:

- o Sweet herbs: these herbs include rose-scented geranium, stevia, lavender, pineapple sage, peppermint, pineapple mint, apple mint, and cinnamon basil, among others.

- o Blossom herbs and spices – Combine basil (10 grams), chili flakes (926 gm), oregano (21 gm), and thyme (22 gm).

The Amber or Oriental family

Most perfumers recommend this fragrance family as it is considered the most luxurious of all. The scents used in this family must have full, rich, sugary, lush, spicy, and aromatic scents.

Just like in the last fragrance family we have discussed, this too has several sub-families. They include:

- **Ambery scents**

  The scents in this sub-family are musky. So, for herbal purposes, use oud (also known as agarwood), amber, and jasmine, among others.

- **Soft ambery**

  The scents you use in this sub-section should be light, and if you want to blend those notes, do so with anise and floral scents.

- **Woody ambery**

  The scents to be used in this subsection should be earthy, sweet, or blended with creamy and smooth earthy patchouli or creamy sandalwood.

The Woody Family

This fragrance wheel family consists of warm, opulent, buttery, rich amber, powdery sandalwood, and sugary cedar scents. Kindly note that woody scents have some level of sweetness, so we recommend blending them with fresh and floral notes.

The Woody family consists of:

- Wood scents consist of patchouli and sandalwood.

- Mossy woods consist of smooth, earthy, and mellow scents such as coffee rubs, achiote, turmeric, lavender, vanilla, lemongrass, ylang-ylang, jasmine, and cumin, among others.

- Dry woods feature smoky notes such as opoponax, styrax, labdanum, cade, and creamy sandalwood notes.

- Aromatic scents- These consist of fresh aromatic, and woody scents such as lavender, cedarwood, vetiver, patchouli, pine, sandalwood, rosemary, mint, and sage, among others.

Now that you know what exactly each section of the fragrance wheel consists of, it is time to learn how to use it. To do so, follow the tips below:

- Always consult your scent notes or what is better yet known as a pyramid.

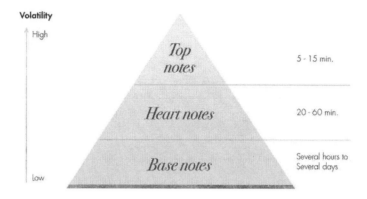

Remember how we discussed the three notes? It is time to use this information. Always pick three scents that complete the whole pyramid. This way, your scents will complement each other without worrying about the aroma being irritating.

- If you are having issues knowing which scents are perfect for the pyramid, you can select scents directly from the fragrance wheel. All you have to do is, choose scents that are side by side only. So, if you pick scents from the floral family, blend them with the opposite scents, which are scents from the woody family.

So, from all we have talked about, let us look at a few examples of scents that complement each other well.

Scent 1: The Ambery Family

- Top notes: bergamot, cardamom, raspberry, and eucalyptus.

- Middle notes: violet, rose, vanilla, and white tea.

- Leg notes: cashmere, cedar wood, and sandalwood.

Scent 2: The Fresh Family

- Head notes: citron, bergamot, pomelo, and sea salt.

- Middle notes: violet, jasmine, and sea moss.

- Leg notes: driftwood and ambergris.

The Floral Family

- Head notes: citrus and orange.

- Heart notes: jasmine, rose, and honeysuckle.

- Leg note: sandalwood

The Woody Family

- Head notes: banana, cardamom, violet, iris, and leafy green.

- Heart notes: cinnamon and apple.

- Leg notes: patchouli and sandalwood.

Binding Agent

A binding agent or a binder is a glue that helps hold the incense together in any shape desired and helps solidify the shape.

There are several types of binders that you can choose from:

- Wood binders

- Plant extract, resins, or gum binders

- Honey binders

From all these binders, there are a few things to note:

- Those who have used honey recommend it because it adds to the overall scent since it has a sweet aroma and it slows down the burning process making the incense last longer.

- Wood binders are also recommended because they are easy to work with, and in most cases, they are also used as incense bases. The best wood binders to use are:

o Joss powder which is also known as jiggit. This binder is viscous and quite adhesive. These two attributes make the incense burn continuously and for a more extended time.

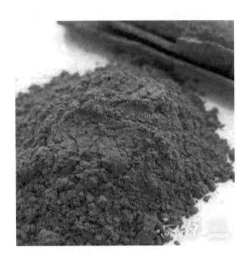

o Tabu no ki, which is also known as makko is perfect for creating different types of incense, such as cylinders, coils, cones, joss sticks, and masala incense sticks, among other shapes. In addition to being versatile, many use it because it is scentless, so you do not have to worry about contaminating your overall fragrance!

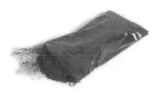

Note:

Be keen when using wood binders because you need to know the right amount to use. All in all, ensure that your recipe has no more than 75 percent wood binder.

- If you would like to use plant extract, resins, or gum binders such as xantham, acacia, almond, aloes, benzoin, loban, copals, dammar, dragon's blood, elemi, fir, maydi, thurifera, beyo-carterii, aden, neglecta, or guar gum, note that they are much stronger as compared to wood binders. So, use no more than an eighth of a teaspoon for every 2 tablespoons of material.

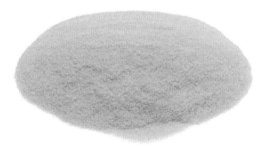

Xantham gum powder

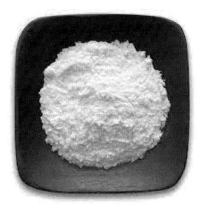

Guar gum powder

If you add more than this, the mixture will be too concentrated that the incense will not burn. On the other side, apart from ensuring that the measurements are right, do not worry about it impacting the incense because it adds no scent of their own to the blend.

Now that we know what incense consists of, it is time to move on to learn how they are made. Let us discuss this next.

Section 2: Tools and Saftey

Apart from what we have discussed so far, you will also need other tools to make your incense. These tools are;

- Measuring scales

- Grinders

- Mortar and pestle

- Incense charcoals

- Burner fillings

- Incense burners

Let us discuss each one of them;

Chapter 4: The Tools and Equipment

Incense Burners

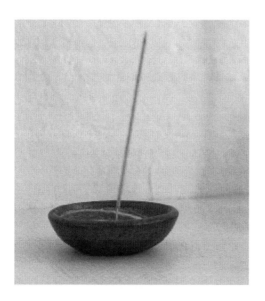

Incense burners might seem optional at this stage, but I believe it is the first tool you should possess because they will help hold your incense while it burns.

Apart from helping hold the incense, they help contain the aroma so that the incense burns evenly and slowly and prevents it from directly contacting the surface because it may damage it by smoke or heat.

Incense burners come in different shapes and sizes. My personal favorite is the backflow incense burners.

Backflow burners are becoming popular because they are designed in such a way that they produce a 'backflow effect.' This effect makes the incense burner's smoke cascade in different ways. An example is the one below;

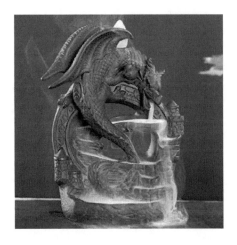

Incense Burner Fillings

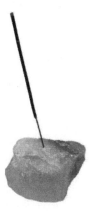

This tool will help insulate the burners. So, to use it, pour some filling in the hole where the incense will sit, then fix into the sit and ignite the incense!

There are four main filler types; salt, crushed rock, sand, and white ash.

I use two types - *ash* because it allows better air circulation and *white chaff filler* because it is versatile, given that you can use it with all kinds of incense.

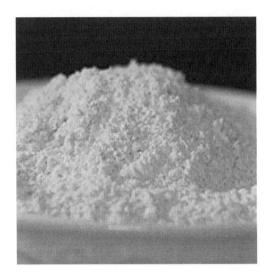

White chaff filler for incense burners

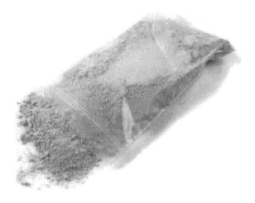

White ash filler for incense burners

Before fixing the incense, kindly remember to add your filler to around half to three-quarters full.

Note:

You can use your incense burner without a filler, especially if you are not using any base material. In this case, I recommend using incense charcoal – place it in the middle of the burner, then sprinkle incense right next to it or on top of it.

Incense Charcoal

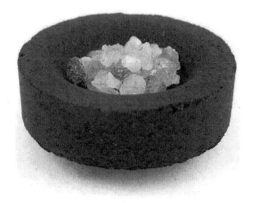

This is a self-combusting material made from compressed coconut shells. Incense charcoal will make combustion possible if you are especially dealing with incense that does not ignite on its own such as herbs and pure tree resins. In addition to helping ignition, incense charcoal helps the charcoal burn off evenly.

Note:

Most self-lighting incense charcoals contain saltpeter and Sulphur, which are toxic chemicals (you will notice such components in your charcoal if it produces strong odors or sparkles after being ignited).

With this in mind, I recommend using chemical-free natural charcoal made using natural roots or bamboo.

Tweezers

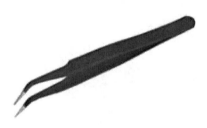

These will help you safely handle charcoals when lighting them and transferring them to the incense burners.

Mortar and Pestle

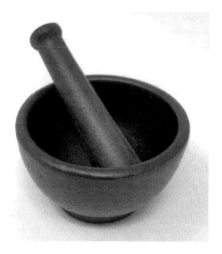

This pair will help you grind your powders and resins to finer particles.

Depending on the amount of incense you want in general or the amount of base you will be grinding at a time, the following are some of the factors that you shoulder before purchasing any mortar and pestle;

- **The size**

Here, decide if you want a mortar that fits single or multiple herbs. In addition to the ingredients in question, size raises the question of safety. Large mortars with small widths tend to harm the hand because you end up hitting it from the side.

So, if you want to use huge mortars, get one that has a big diameter on top.

- **The shape**

You might find some mortars with different corners such as bumps or other features outside of the mortar but in as much as this might seem artistic, purchase one with a round shape and no corners at all because this will make grinding much easier.

- **The material**

Since you might be grinding woody herbs most of the time, which means doing a lot of pounding and grinding, you need a pestle and mortar that is strong enough. This means purchasing one made from materials such as marble and granite. Do not purchase mortars and pestles made from wood, light metal, or weak ceramic materials because they are not strong enough to handle the pressure.

With these factors in mind, let us look at some of the mortars and pestles with the attributes we have just discussed;

- **Thai granite mortars and pestles**

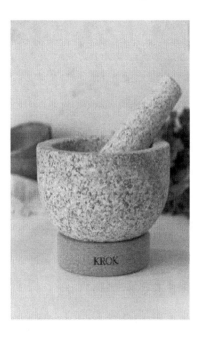

As the name suggests, these mortars and pestles are made from solid granite,, which means they can handle both soft and tough herbs. The bottom of these mortars have corks that help dampen the noise created while grinding and pounding.

The Italian marble mortars with wood pestles

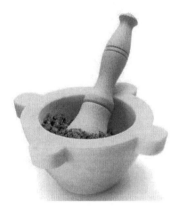

The granite mortar and pestle can grind down woody and other tough herbs into fine powder, but this type of mortar and pestle does an even finer job. You can therefore use the granite mortar and pestle to break down the tough herbs, then transfer the powder to this mortar and use its pestle to get that finer texture.

- ## The Japanese mortar and pestle

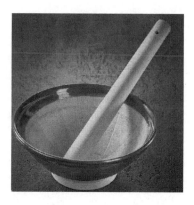

This mortar has cut ridges inside, which pushes the herbs downwards as a fine powder or paste if you grind materials such as rose buds or petals, among others. If you decide to purchase this mortar and pestle, choose a mortar with ridges that go in two directions because you can work with it left-handed or right-handed.

Note:

Once done using your mortar and pestle, wash them with a mixture of water and soap (use unscented soap). You can choose to rub it with a dishrag or soft cloth.

You can also use the following tools to grind your herbs and binding agents;

Electric spice grinders

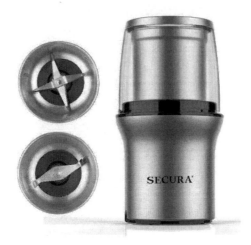

- **Grinding food processer**

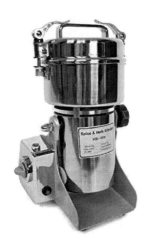

- **Manual coffee grinder**

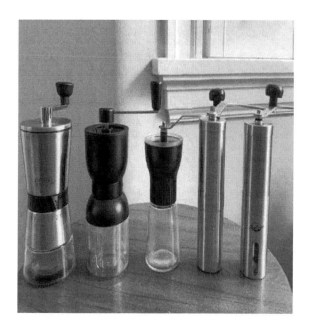

- **Rasp grater**

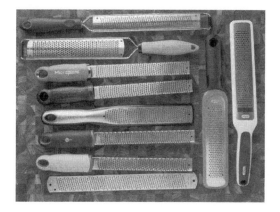

- **Rolling pin**

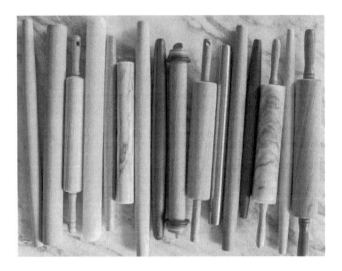

Measuring Spoons and Scales

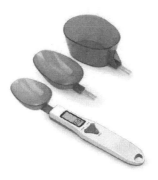

Measuring spoon

- **Measuring scale**

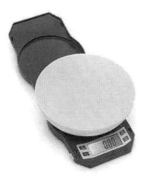

These scales will help you know the exact binding agent and liquid to use depending on the amount of base material that you will use. Purchase a scale that measures as little as 0.1 grams because you will mostly deal with grams.

If you prefer to measure by spoon, improve your accuracy by purchasing a measuring spoon that is calibrated or attached to a digital measurement scale.

Once you get your tools ready, it is time to protect yourself. Let us learn how next.

Chapter 5: Incense Safety Precautions

As you work on creating your own incense, please keep the following factors into consideration.

Handle With Care

If you are making incense from home, do not leave the essential oils lying around because some are toxic if consumed in high amounts by humans and pets.

These essential oils include;

- Wintergreen

- Verbena

- Rosemary

- Peppermint

- Fennel

- Eucalyptus

...among others.

So, generally, when handling essential oils, keep the following things in mind;

- **Dilute essential oils**

Always dilute all essential oils before use, although some experts say that Lavandula angustifolia (English lavender), Chamaemelum nobile (Roman chamomile), helichrysum italicum (curry plant), cypress, tea tree, rose and melaleuca alternifolia (narrow-leaved paperbark) can be used undiluted.

This will lower their concentration levels. I recommend diluting essential oils with a few drops of carrier oils (these oils are also made from plants), such as;

- o Black seed oil

- o Rosehip oil

- o Argan oil

- o Olive oil

- o Sweet almond oil

- o Apricot kernel oil

- o Jojoba oil

- Coconut oil

- **Regularly do a patch test**

This is a test that is used to detect the presence or absence of skin rashes or skin allergies that essential oils might cause. To do a patch test, follow the steps below;

- First, after contact with any essential oils, wash your hands or the place that has come in contact with the oils. I recommend doing the washing with soap and water too.

- After washing properly, pat dry.

- Drop a few drops of the essential oils on the forearm, put a gauze, then wait for 24 hours

- After 24 hours, remove the gauze, then assess the forearm

If your skin turns red, itchy, or swollen, or if you notice some blistering, this is an indicator that the essential is too concentrated, so consider diluting it more.

Once diluted, do another patch test, and if the same symptoms present themselves, consider changing the oil because you might be allergic to it.

With all this information in mind, the following are the essential oils that **must** be diluted;

- o Bay oil

- o Thyme oil

- o Oregano oil

- o Lemon verbena oil

- o Lemongrass oil

- o Cumin oil

- o Citronella oil

- o Clove bud oil

- o Cinnamon bark or leaf oil

The following are some of the essential oils that do not need diluting;

- o Sandalwood oil
- o Rose oil
- o Tea tree oil
- o Lavender oil
- o Eucalyptus oil
- o Cypress oil
- o Chamomile oil

If you are pregnant or if you are breastfeeding, do not use the following types of essential oils because their toxicity levels are too high;

- o Wormwood oil
- o Wintergreen oil
- o Tarragon oil
- o Pennyroyal oil
- o Hyssop oil

o   Parsley seed

o   Camphor oil

The following oils should not be used around infants and children because their bodies cannot handle the potency!

o   Wintergreen oil

o   Verbena oil

o   Rosemary oil

o   Peppermint oil

o   Fennel oil

o   Eucalyptus oil

Ventilate Your Workspace

Numerous studies have affirmed that the smoke released by incense might be toxic and hazardous to health. Suppose you do not properly ventilate your workspace. In that case, there are high chances you will suffer from[5] changes in lung cell

---

[5]   https://sph.unc.edu/sph-news/151807-2/#:~:text=Previous%20studies%2C%20some%20by%20Yeatts,changes%20in%20lung%20cell%20structure.

structure, cardiovascular illnesses, headaches, asthma, dermatitis, throat, nose, and eye irritation.

So, before making any incense;

Ensure your room is well-ventilated. If the space has poor wall ventilators or a small number of openings, purchase an air purifier or move your workspace outside.

Only Use Herbs Approved by the Food and Drug Administration

In the US, the Food and Drug Administration has the full list of the herbs you should use. The following are some of the approved herbs[6];

Certainly! Here's the list reshuffled:

• Passionflower

• Licorice root

• Green tea

• Flaxseed and flaxseed oil

• Grape seed extract

---

[6] **https://www.nccih.nih.gov/health/herbsataglance**

- St. John's wort

- Aloe vera

- Ginger

- Rhodiola

- Red clover

- Milk thistle

- Saw palmetto

- Sage

- Black cohosh

- Cranberry

- Pomegranate

- Echinacea

- Tea tree oil

- Turmeric

- Soy

- Ginkgo

- Garlic

- Bilberry

- Hawthorn

- Acai

- Bromelain

- Evening primrose oil

- Chasteberry

- Astragalus

- Goldenseal

- Valerian

- Asian ginseng

- Chamomile

- Feverfew

- Yohimbe

- Dandelion

- Noni

- Butterbur

- Kava

- European mistletoe

- Thunder God vine

- Mugwort

- Bitter orange

- Cat's claw

The following are some of the <u>unapproved herbs</u>[7];

- Ma huang

- Licorice

- Germander

- Chaparral

- Sassafras

- Life root

[7]
<u>**https://pubmed.ncbi.nlm.nih.gov/10030529/#:~:text=Many%2 0herbs%20have%20been%20identified,John's%20wort%2C%2 0and%20valerian**</u>.

- Comfrey

- Coltsfoot

- Calamus

- Borage

With all this in mind, if you encounter an unfamiliar herb, you can check if it is approved through the FDA database[8].

Blend Your Fragrances The Right Way

You might be content with a single fragrance such as juniper, but this should not be a reason to block out some adventure. Blending fragrances is a fun way of creating your own signature fragrance by drawing notes from different oils and adding them to the new fragrance.

There are several ways to group essential oils;

Blending Essential Oils by Note

Earlier in this book, while discussing how scents should are classified into notes, we mentioned and discussed three types of notes – head, heart, or legs. We said that the scents from

---

[8]   https://www.fda.gov/industry/fda-basics-industry/search-databases#search-form

the head are the lightest, and they are the first ones you will smell. These scents should be citrusy or floral.

For the head notes, you can try;

- Sage

- Spearmint

- Eucalyptus

- Basil

- Pine needle

- Petitgrain

- Sweet orange

- Lime

- Lemongrass

- Lemon

- Grapefruit

- Citronella

- Bergamot

The middle notes, which we mentioned as the heart, should be a scent that binds the head and the legs. To identify what scents to use for this category, use oils from whole herbs and spices.

For the heart notes, you can try;

- Red thyme

- Tea tree

- Rosemary

- Oregano

- Marjoram

- Clary sage

- Chamomile

- Juniper berry

- Cypress

- Nutmeg

- Clove

- Cinnamon leaf

- Coriander

- Palmarosa

- Geranium

- Rose geranium

- Lavender

The leg notes, which are considered the base notes, should be deeper, meaning they should be heavier. They should not only be heavy but blend with the head scents to help it last longer, even after the incense burns out. These scents should be from woody herbs.

For the leg notes, you can try;

- Peppermint

- Vetiver

- Sandalwood

- Patchouli

- Frankincense

- Cedarwood atlas

- Black pepper

- Ylang ylang

Blending Essential Oils by Fragrance

Before you blend any fragrance, let us go back a bit and group all the known fragrances. To do this, we will group them into 5 main categories which are;

- **Woody fragrance**

In this category, we have the following fragrance scents;

- Birch scent

- Gaiac scent

- Oud scent

- Cypress scent

- Vetiver scent

- Patchouli scent

- Cedar scent

- Sandalwood scent

- **Spicy fragrance**

In this category, we have the following fragrance scents;

- o Juniper scent

- o Ginger scent

- o Timut pepper scent

- o Pink pepper scent

- o Coriander scent

- o Cardamon scent

- **Herbal fragrance**

In this category, we have the following fragrance scents;

- o Neroli scent

- o Rose scent

- o Vetiver scent

- o Sandalwood scent

- o Cinnamon orange clove scent

- o Amber scent

- **Floral fragrance**

In this category, we have the following fragrance scents;

- o Neroli scent

- o Gardenia scent

- o Tuberose scent

- o Orange blossom scent

- o Lily of the valley scent

- o Jasmine scent

○ Rose scent

- **Citrus fragrance**

In this category, we have the following fragrance scents;

    ○ Yuzu scent

    ○ Grapefruit scent

    ○ Neroli scent

    ○ Bergamot scent

    ○ Lime scent

    ○ Orange scent

These five categories can go hand in hand with the following fragrances;

Citrus – This category blends with scents such as spicy, herbal, and floral scents. This means that you can blend spicy scents with the following scents;

- Sweet orange scent

- Neroli scent

- Lime scent

- Lemongrass scent

- Lemon scent

- Grapefruit scent

- Citronella scent

- Bergamot scent

On the other hand, the following scents do not complement citrus;

- Peppermint

- Thyme

- Basil

- Ylang ylang

- Jasmine

- Rosemary blends

- Patchouli

- Lemon essential oils

Woody – This category blends with spicy, herbal, citrus, and floral scents. This means that you can blend spicy scents with the following scents;

- Red thyme scent

- Tea tree scent

- Sage scent

- Rosemary scent

- Oregano scent

- Spearmint scent

- Marjoram scent

- Eucalyptus scent

- Clary sage scent

- Chamomile scent

- Basil scent

Do not mix woody scents with oriental scents. These include scents such as;

- Ambergris

- Vanilla

- Tonka bean

- Patchouli

- Benzoin balm

- Peruvian balsam

- Myrrh

- Styrax

- Cloves

- Cinnamon

Spicy - This category blends with citrus, woody, and floral scents. This means that you can blend spicy scents with the following scents;

- Vetiver scent

- Scandal wood scent

- Pine needle scent

- Petitgrain scent

- Patchouli scent

- Juniper berry scent

- Frankincense scent

- Cypress scent

- Cedarwood atlas scent

Now that you know which fragrances can blend, I strongly recommend choosing oils from the same families first, then blending equal amounts of each fragrance (you can blend fragrances from different categories as you advance or as you start to recognize different scents and develop a niche).

You can start with the following fragrance blends;

- Sweet orange/grapefruit/lemon/peppermint

- Lavender/geranium/sandalwood

Blending Essential Oils by Effect

To blend essential oils, start by looking at their properties. So, in this case, it is important to know the benefits of each herb.

Let me give you some examples;

- **Rosemary** – this herb will boost[9] your body's antibacterial, antifungal, and antiviral systems to enhance the body's immune system and lower the risks of diseases and infection.

- **Parsley**– this herb will help reduce blood pressure[10] and bloating[11] , meaning it is a potent diuretic.

- **Oregano** – this herb is rich in antioxidants, helps fight bacteria[12], and reduces cancerous properties[13], viral infection[14], and inflammation[15].

- **Mint** – this herb is known, to some extent, to improve irritable bowel syndrome, which reduces digestive tract disorders.[16]

- **Dill** – this herb will help reduce the risk of stroke and heart diseases and disorders[17].

---

[9] https://www.ncbi.nlm.nih.gov/pmc/articles/PMC7491497/

[10]   https://healthmatch.io/high-blood-pressure/can-herbs-help-high-blood-pressure

[11] https://scholar.google.com/scholar?as_ylo=2019&q=+parsley+reduces+bloating&hl=en&as_sdt=0,5

[12] **https://www.mdpi.com/2076-0817/8/1/15**

[13] **https://www.ncbi.nlm.nih.gov/pmc/articles/PMC6508890/**

[14] https://ijisrt.com/assets/upload/files/IJISRT21AUG251.pdf

[15] https://www.mdpi.com/2297-8739/8/12/240

[16] https://link.springer.com/article/10.1007/s10620-019-05523-8

- **Cilantro** – this herb [helps reduce heart disease][18], [obesity][19], [diabetes][20], and [seizures][21].

- **Basil** – this may help reduce depression and anxiety, boosts your ability to think, and [lowers dementia and other age-related memory loss illnesses and disorders][22].

If categorizing in this manner seems challenging, you can also organize them into 4 main groups:

- **Grounding oils** – these oils will help calm you down and make you more aware. The most common herbs that produce grounding oils are;

    o Red thyme

---

[17] https://www.indianjournals.com/ijor.aspx?target=ijor:ajrps&volume=10&issue=4&article=003

[18] https://pubs.acs.org/doi/abs/10.1021/acs.jafc.2c00267

[19] https://pubs.acs.org/doi/abs/10.1021/acs.jafc.2c00267

[20] https://cyberleninka.ru/article/n/coriander-for-health-what-scientists-say-about-the-benefits-and-harms-of-seasoning

[21] https://www.researchgate.net/profile/Gaurav-Saxena-19/publication/361984196 International Journal of Botany Studies wwwbotanyjournalscom Evaluation of anti-epileptic activity of Coriandrum sativum fruit extracts/links/62cfe3 257156f534a6825d80/International-Journal-of-Botany-Studies-wwwbotanyjournalscom-Evaluation-of-anti-epileptic-activity-of-Coriandrum-sativum-fruit-extracts.pdf

[22] https://link.springer.com/article/10.1007/s11356-021-17830-7

- o Spearmint

- o Marjoram

- o Chamomile

- o Vetiver

- o Sandalwood

- o Frankincense

- o Cedarwood atlas

- o Oregano

- o Clove

- o Black pepper

- o Coriander

- o Lavender

- o Geranium

- o Rose geranium

- o Sweet orange

- o Bergamot

- **Cleansing oils** – these herbs cleanse the body and mind. The most common herbs that produce cleansing oils are;

    o Peppermint

    o Patchouli

    o Juniper berry

    o Oregano

    o Nutmeg

    o Sweet orange

    o Lime

    o Lemon

    o Grapefruit

    o Citronella

- **Relaxing oils** – these oils will help you unwind. The following herbs will produce these oils;

    o Red thyme

    o Sage

- o Clary sage

- o Vetiver

- o Patchouli

- o Frankincense

- o Cedarwood atlas

- o Nutmeg

- o Ylang ylang

- o Palmarosa

- o Lavender

- o Geranium

- o Roe geranium

- o Bergamot

- **Energizing oils** – these oils will help refresh your mind. Use them to kickstart your day. The following are the herbs that produce these oils;

  - o Tea tree

  - o Sage

- Rosemary
- Peppermint
- Spearmint
- Eucalyptus
- Clary sage
- Basil
- Pine needle
- Petitgrain
- Cypress
- Clove
- Cinnamon leaf
- Black pepper
- Coriander
- Sweet orange
- Lime
- Lemongrass

- o Lemon

- o Grapefruit

- o Citronella

- o Bergamot

You can start by blending oils from one category first; then, as you get accustomed to the different scents, you can combine different categories.

With this said, the following are good examples of blends by effect;

- Lemon/grapefruit/peppermint (this is from the energizing oils category)

- Bergamot/patchouli/ylang-ylang (this is from the relaxing oils category)

Now that you have your tools ready and are certain about which incense you want to make, let us create 50 of the most common and uncommon herbal recipes known today!

Let us do this next.

Section 4: The Recipes

Chapter 6: Herbal Incense Recipes

Note:

There are different ways of making incense. However, the following are the most standard ways of making incense, which can be used as general guidelines for the recipes that will follow:

Standard Ways of Making Herbal Incense

1. Smudge incense

To create smudge incense using your favorite herbs, follow the steps below:

Materials Required

- Herbs

- Scissors

- Cotton string or any string made from natural materials

- Hanger

Procedure

- First, gather your favorite herbs and set them up in a bundle.

- Tie your bundle using cotton string then secure the base with a knot.

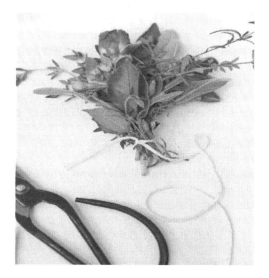

- From the base, crisscross the bundle using the cotton string. Do not make the wrapping too tight, as this may crush the herbs.

- Use your scissors to cut off the excess string.

- Hand the wrapped bundle upside down in a cool, dry place for at least seven days.

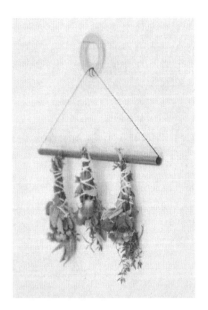

- After the bundle dries, your incense is ready! All that is left to do is, place the bundle in a bowl, then light it from one end.

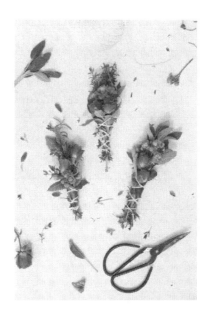

2. Loose incense

This type of incense is made from loose-leaf herbs, resins, and bits of bark. Unlike stick or cone incense, they are not made from any additives that help them burn continuously. This, therefore, means you will always need a constant heat source if you are to create loose incense.

To make your loose incense, follow the basic steps below:

Materials Required

- Constant heat source such as charcoal discs, heat proof bowls, tongs, sand/ash/rocks/beans, and lighters

- Herbs

- Resins

- Bark bits

Procedure

- First, prepare the heat bowl. To do this, add some sand/ash/salt to the bowl first.

- Add an already-heated charcoal disc.

- Finally, after the charcoal becomes hot, sprinkle the loose herbs, bark, and resins on top.

3. Stick and Cone incense

These two types of cones are made rather the same way but are formed in two main shapes: cones or sticks

To make them, follow the steps below:

Materials Required

- Herbs

- Mortar and pestle

- Water and/or any other liquid ingredients

- Piping tip

- Straw

Procedure

- First, choose your herbs, then grind them using a mortar and pestle.

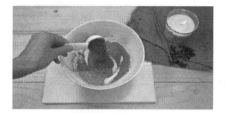

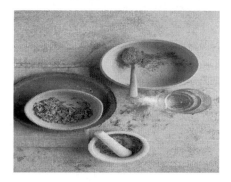

- Add your liquid as per the number of herbs you have ground.

- Mold the mixture into either sticks or cones. For sticks, you can use a straw to ensure it's straight and the same size; for cones use a piping tip.

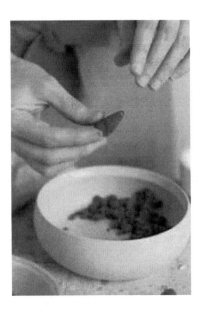

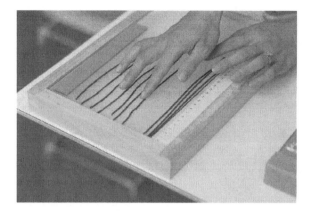

- Finally, dry the incense, and you should be ready to burn them!

You can use the three ways we have discussed above to create any of the following incense:

Incense Recipe 1

In this recipe, we will learn how to make juniper-scented incense.

Base: Dry Juniper Powder

Liquid: Water

Color: Brown

Bonding Agent: Makko powder or what is known as tabu no ki powder

Other Materials Required

- Grinder or pestle and mortar

- Spoon

- Container

- Water

- Incense blanks

- Matchbox

Procedure

- Grind the juniper particles till they are fine.

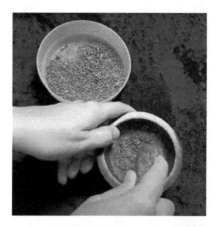

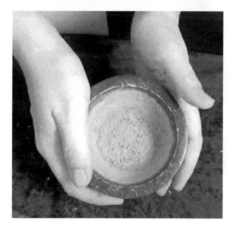

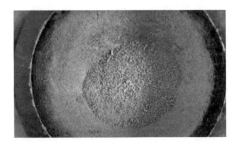

- After grinding, measure your juniper powder (the total came to 2 and a half tablespoons).

- Pour makko powder into a separate bowl (this recipe measured 2 tablespoons).

- Pour the juniper powder into a separate bowl, then mix thoroughly.

- Add some water. Follow the instructions that came with the binding agent to know just how much water to add.

- Knead the mixture as you continue adding water (Do not add too much water at a time).

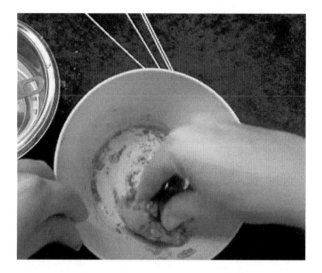

- Knead it till it gets a bread dough consistency. Once done, feel the dough. If it is sticky, add some makko powder, then continue kneading.

- The dough should resemble the image below.

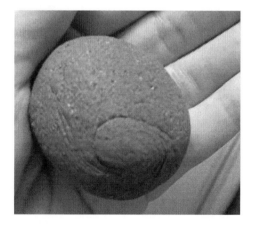

- Once the dough is ready, it is time to wrap it around the incense blanks. To do this, roll the dough into the size and length of the blanks. Look at the image below;

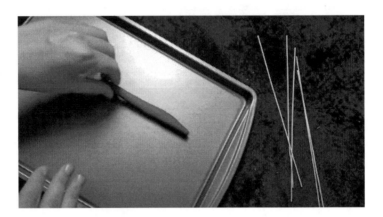

- Once the rolled dough satisfies you, take a blank and press it on the dough. Then roll the dough around the blank.

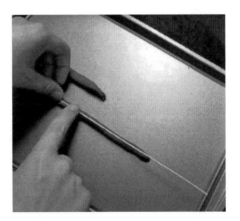

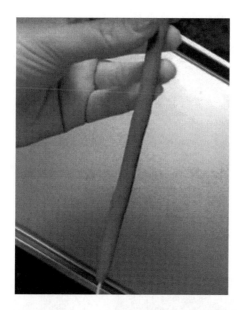

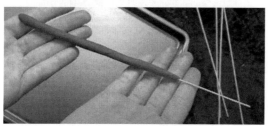

- Make as many stick incenses as you can. You can make different shapes with the sticks. Below is a cone shape.

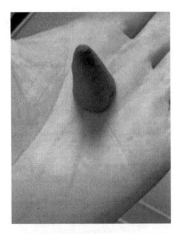

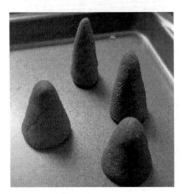

- Once your dough is all wrapped in one way or another around the blanks, let the incense dry for at least 48 hours.

- Test the incense sticks and cones out.

- If you have a cone that is not wrapped around a blank, burn the tip, then fan it out.

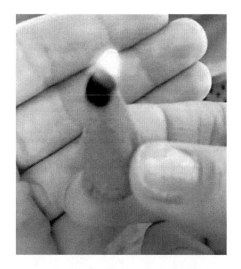

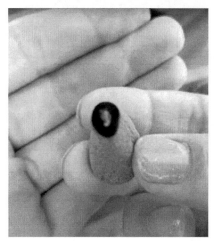

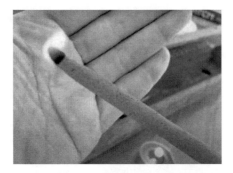

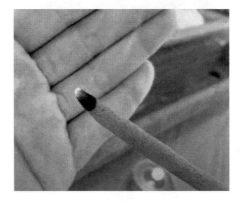

Finally, let one burn all way to check if you have done everything right, and you're done!

Incense Recipe 2

In this recipe, we will learn how to make blended scented incense. We will use 5 different bases to create a new scent.

Base: Dry rose flower, dry orange peels, clove/lavangam, cardamon/elakkai, sandalwood/Chandan

Liquid: Water

Bonding Agent: Cinnamon powder, edible camphor, and benzoin resin powder/sambrani powder

Other Materials Required

- Sieve

- Grinder

- Spoon

- Container

- Sambrani cone die mold

Procedure

- Get your dry rose flower, dry orange peels, clove/lavangam, cardamon/elakkai, and sandalwood/Chandan then grind them together. Ensure that the grind produces a fine powder.

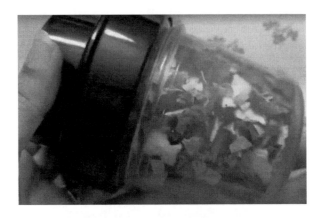

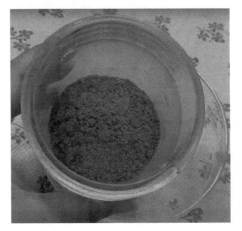

- Sieve the powder into a separate container.

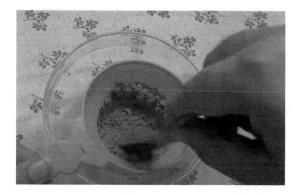

- Add the cinnamon powder, then mix well.

- Add edible champor/pachi karpooram, then mix well.

- Add benzoin resin powder/sambrani powder, then mix again.

- Add water to the mixture, then mix till it turns into large particles

- Take a piece of plastic paper, then shape it into a cone. To keep the shape together, seal it with a bit of tape.

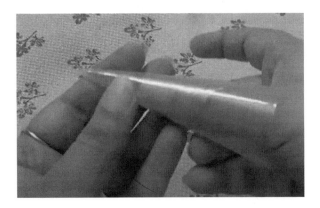

- Fill the cone with the mixture.

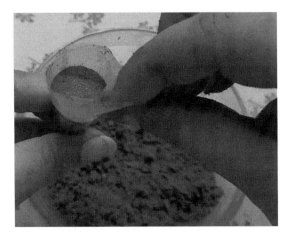

- After pressing the mixture down, slide it out of the plastic-shaped-cone.

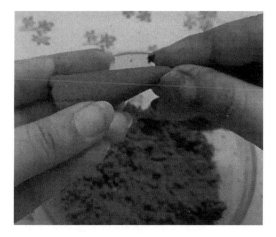

- After you are done making your cones, let them dry well.

- You can also use a sambrani cone die mold to make the cones. To do this, fill the mold with the mixture.

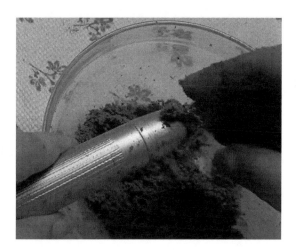

- This is the shape the mold is used to produce.

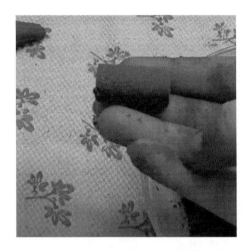

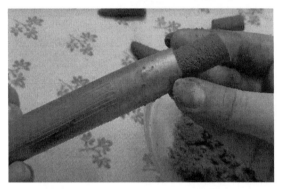

- After your cones are dry, they are ready for burning.

Incense Recipe 3

In this recipe, we will learn how to make blended scented incense. We will use 8 different bases to create a new scent.

Base: Ginger root, peppermint or piperita, bupleurum root, Bai zhu, atractylodes, white peony root, charcoal, and dong quai

Liquid: Water

Bonding Agent: Licorice root, makko, and vitamix

Note:

Use any of the discussed standard methods to create this incense.

Incense Recipe 4

In this recipe, we will learn how to make blended scented incense. We will use 8 different bases to create a new scent.

Base: Bayberry root, mandrake, meadowsweet, myrrh, penny royal, red sandalwood, and vervain.

Other required materials

- Mortar and pestle
- Coal diskettes
- Lighter
- Tongs

Procedure

- Use a mortar and pestle to grind bayberry root, then put it in a different container.
- Grind the mandrake, then add it to the container. The amount of mandrake should be less than bayberry.
- Grind meadowsweet, then add it to the container
- Grind the myrrh, then add it to the container.

- Grind the penny royal, then add it to the container

- Grind the red sandalwood, then add it to the container.

- Grind the vervain, then add it to the container.

- Warmup the coal diskettes.

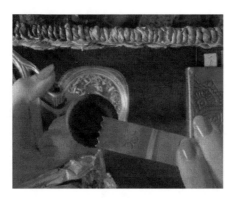

- Finally, pour the mixture into the diskette and enjoy your incense!

Incense Recipe 5

In this recipe, we will learn how to make white sage-scented incense.

Base: White sage

Liquid: Water

Bonding Agent: Makko powder

Other required materials

- Mortar and pestle

- Spoon

- Container

- Twist tie

- A board lined with wax paper

- Sun or fan

- Sand

Procedure

- Grind sage using mortar and pestle

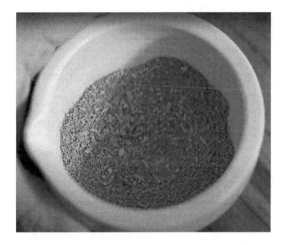

- Measure three teaspoons of the powdered sage and put it in a separate.

- Add water with a dropper to make a dough.

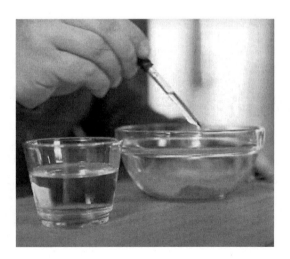

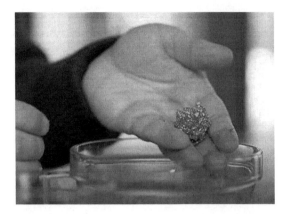

- Take conical-shaped metal tips (these are typically attached to icing bags for cake decorations), then fill them with the dough.

- To remove the molded cone, slip a twist tie into the tip.

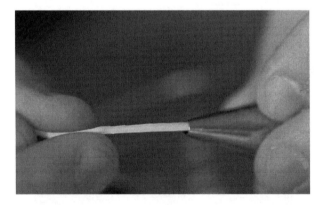

- Since the shaped incense has not yet dried up, lay it on a board line with wax paper.

- Lay the cones in the sun or a fan to dry. If you use the fan, set it on a 'low setting to dry. After 12 hours, lay them on their side. This will make it possible for them to dry all around.

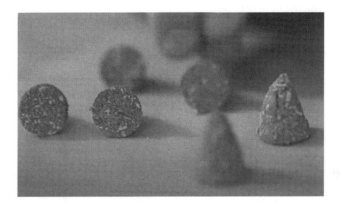

- Fill another container (the container should be heat-resistant) with sand, then lay your burning cone, and you are done!

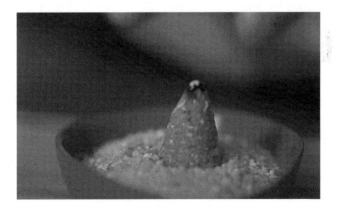

Incense Recipe 6

In this recipe, we will learn how to make blended scented incense. We will use 2 different bases to create a new scent.

Base: Lavender and sandalwood

Liquid: Lavender tea and lavender essential oil

Bonding Agent: Copal resin and makko powder

Note:

Use any of the discussed standard methods to create this incense.

Incense Recipe 7

In this recipe, we will learn how to make blended scented incense. We will use 2 different bases to create a new scent.

Base: Lavender and sandalwood

Essential Oil: Geranium essential oil

Bonding Agent: White copal, honey, and dragon's blood

Other materials required

- Containers

- Mortar and pestle

- Incense burner

- Charcoal disks

- Tongs

- Foil paper

- Candle

- Sieve

- Candle container

- Foil paper

Procedure

- Grind white copal and dragon's blood using a mortar and pestle.

- Add all the other bases to the container with the resins.

- Stir everything well with a spoon.

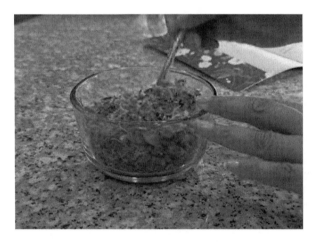

- Add geranium oil.

- Add honey.

- Stir everything together nicely.

- Depending on how much consistency you want the mixture to have, add more honey as you continue stirring. Just be keen not to make it so sticky because it will not burn well.

- Set up your incense burner and charcoal.

- Light up the charcoal disks. Hold them using your pair of tongs.

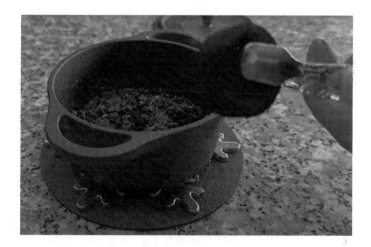

- Put your incense mixture in the pot.

- Pour some incense on the disk.

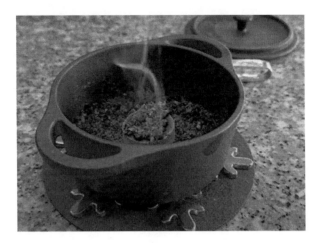

- You can also use a tea light incense warmer. It looks like the one below;

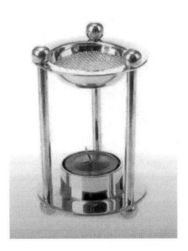

- This is a candle holder with a sieve on top. So, put a candle inside and the incense on top of the sieve. Before you pour the incense into the sieve, line it with foil paper.

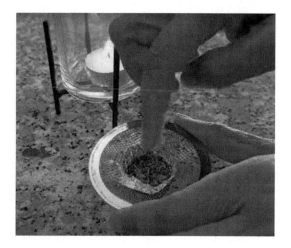

- And your incense is ready!

Incense Recipe 8

In this recipe, we will learn how to make lavender-scented incense.

Base: French lavender oil

Bonding Agent: Di Propylene Glyco

Note:

Use any of the discussed standard methods to create this incense.

Incense Recipe 9

In this recipe, we will learn how to make blended scented incense. We will use 9 different bases to create a new scent.

Base: pumpkin pie spice, ginger, nutmeg, clove, rose petals, bay, sage, rosemary, and cinnamon

Liquid: Water

Bonding Agent: Makko powder

Note:

Use any of the discussed standard methods to create this incense.

Incense Recipe 10

In this recipe, we will learn how to make pine-scented incense.

Base: Pine resin

Other Materials Required

- Scraper

- A piece of a saucer to place the resin

- Lighter

- Soapstone incense burner

- Spoon

Procedure

- Scrap the bark of a pine tree. The aim is to get the whitish product. This will be our pine resin.

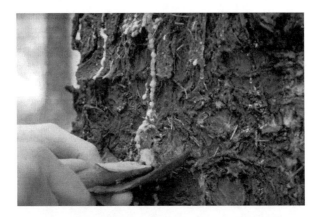

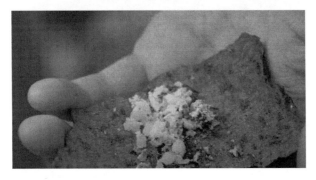

- Remove any pine needles, yellow bits, or bark bits from the resin.

- Burn the resin using a soapstone oil burner. To do this, warm up the oil burner, then pour a few pieces on top.

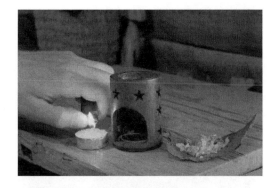

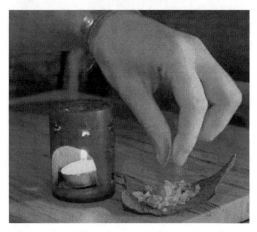

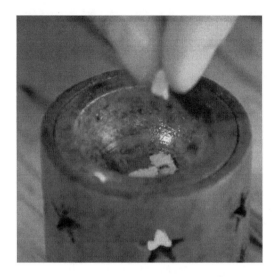

- As the burner warms, the resin will melt, producing a vapor.

- You can also burn the resin with a spoon. Do not use a kitchen spoon because it will char.

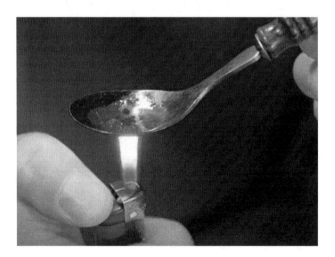

Incense Recipe 11

In this recipe, we will learn how to make blended scented incense. We will use 2 different bases to create a new scent.

Base: frankincense and lavender essential oils

Bonding Agent: Glycol oil

Other Materials Required

- Baking trays

- Unscented incense sticks

- Lighter or matchbox

Procedure

- Mix one-third of the fragrance oils and two-thirds of the glycol oil into one container, giving the two liquids a good mix. Be keen about the measurements, especially of the bonding agent, because too much of it will produce black smoke when burned.

- Soak the unscented incense sticks in the mixed fragrance oils.

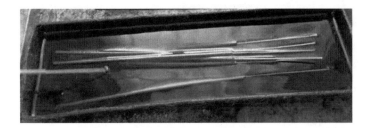

- Once content that they are soaked (you can soak them for 24 hours), lay them on a paper towel, then let them dry out for at least 24 hours or so.

- I soaked them for two days, then let them dry for another 5 days to ensure that the herbal fragrance had been soaked in the sticks properly.

- Once completely dry, your incense sticks are ready to be used!

Incense Recipe 12

In this recipe, we will learn how to make nag champa-scented incense.

Base: Nag champa essential oil

Bonding Agent: DPG (de propylene glycol)

Other Materials Required

- Disposal pipettes – 1 will be for the bonding agent and the other for the nag champa

- Tray

- Unscented incense sticks

Procedure

- Use your pipette to suck some nag champa, then pour it on the tray.

- Use your pipette to suck some DPG, then empty it on the same tray.

- Slightly tilt the tray, then roll up one stick after the other in the accumulated liquid. Look at the images below;

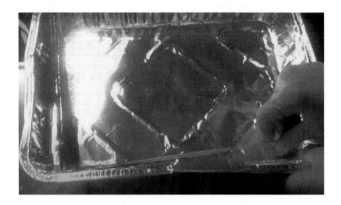

- Finally, let the soaked sticks dry for at least 24 hours, and you are done!

Incense Recipe 13

In this recipe, we will learn how to make blended scented incense. We will use 9 different bases to create a new scent.

Base: neem and thulasi leaves, thulasi and vetiver twigs, scutch grass, cinnamon, nutmeg, licorice root, and white mustard.

Liquid: Rosewater

Bonding Agent: Ghee and camphor

Note:

Use any of the discussed standard methods to create this incense.

Incense Recipe 14

In this recipe, we will learn how to create cannabis incense.

Base: Cannabis essential oil

Note:

Use any of the discussed standard methods to create this incense.

Incense Recipe 15

In this recipe, we will learn how to make blended scented incense. We will use 9 different bases to create a new scent.

We will also learn how to create a backflow incense burner that fits almost every incense cone.

Base: pumpkin pie spice, ginger, nutmeg, clove, rose petals, bay, sage, rosemary, and cinnamon

Liquid: Water

Bonding Agent: Makko powder

Note:

Use any of the discussed standard methods to create this incense.

Incense Recipe 16

In this recipe, we will learn how to make incense from different resins.

Base: frankincense, jasmine, and Cyprus essential oils

Bonding Agent: frankincense resin

Other Materials Required

- Measuring scales

- Spoons

- Bowls

- Resin burner

- Bamboo charcoal

- Incense tongs

- Lighter

Procedure

- Measure an ounce of frankincense.

- Pour 5 drops of frankincense oil into the resin.

- Pour 4 drops of Cyprus oil into the resin.

- Pour 1 drop of jasmine oil into the resin.

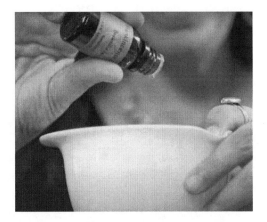

- Mix the ingredients above well using a spoon.

- Hold a piece of bamboo charcoal with the incense tongs, then light it.

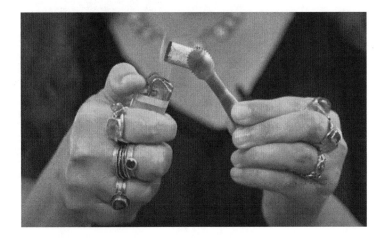

- Place the burning bamboo charcoal in the resin burner.

- Take a pinch or two of the blends we made earlier, then place it in the resin burner.

- Enjoy your incense!

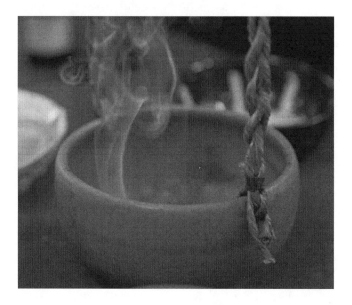

Incense Recipe 17

In this recipe, we will learn how to make Lammas scented incense using 5 bases.

Base: dried marigold or calendula flower petals, sandalwood, oak leaf, rosemary, and rose petals

Bonding Agent: Dragon's blood resin, patchouli essential oil, and honey

Other Materials Required

- Mortar and pestle

- Spoon

- Lighter

- Knife

- Bowl

- Charcoal

- Cast iron cauldron

- Lighter

- Incense tongs

Procedure

- Put some dragon's blood resin in a mortar and pestle, then grind it till it becomes fine.

- Add dried calendula or marigold flower petals to the already ground mixture, then grind it down.

- Add dried sunflower petals to the ground mixture, then grind it down.

- After you are done grinding the herbs above, put them aside in another container.

- Grind some rose petals.

- Add rosemary leaves to the ground rose petals, then continue grinding.

- Add an oak leaf to the ground herbs, then continue grinding.

- Add sandalwood to the ground herbs, then grind. For easier sandalwood grinding, especially if you purchase it in stick form, you might need to slice it with a craft knife or any other type of knife.

- Pour all the ingredients we have worked on into one bowl, then mix with a spoon.

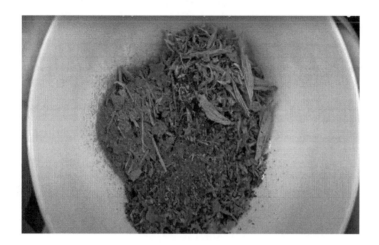

- Add a few drops of patchouli essential oil, then mix with a spoon.

- Add a few drops of rose oil, then mix again.

- Add half a teaspoon of honey, and mix.

- Light some charcoal, then place it in the cast iron cauldron.

- Finally, pour some incense on top of the charcoal, and you will be done!

Incense Recipe 18

In this recipe, we will learn how to make a smudge stick scented incense.

Base: thyme, rosemary, mint, and lavender

Binding agent: Marshmallow root and local honey

Other Materials Required

- Containers or petri dishes

- Spoons

- Mortar and pestle

- Piping cone

- Toothpick

Procedure

- First grind all your bases, then put them in separate containers. Use mortar and pestle for this.

- Measure around 3 tablespoons of each base.

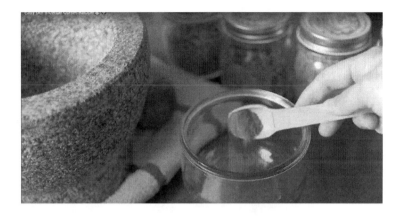

- Mix the grounded herbs thoroughly.

- Grind arrow marshmallow root, then add one tablespoon of marshmallow root powder.

- Mix thoroughly.

- Add 1 tablespoon of water, then continue mixing.

- Add one tablespoon of local honey, then continue mixing.

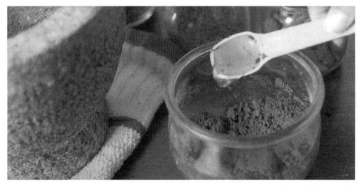

- Mix till you get a dough.

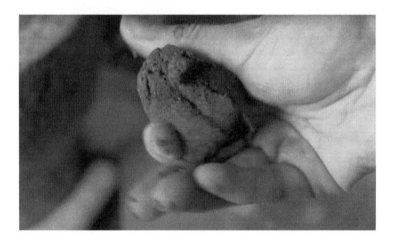

- Take a piping cone and fill it with the dough.

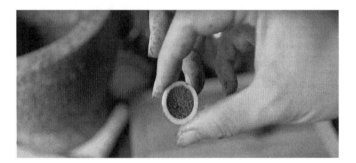

- Take a toothpick and make a hole at the bottom. This will make sure that the incense burns all the way through.

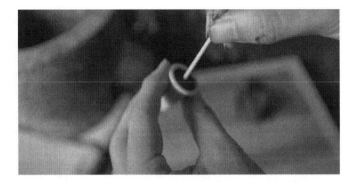

- Overturn the piping cone and tap hard against a flat, sturdy surface till the cone comes off. Then assess it to affirm it's molded correctly.

  If it does not come off, push it out with a toothpick.

- Repeat till you get the number of cones you want.

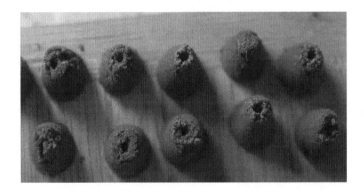

- Finally, allow the incense cones to dry for at least 24 hours, set one on a non-inflammable surface then light it and enjoy!

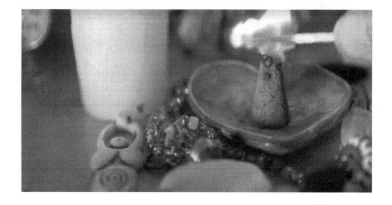

Incense Recipe 19

In this recipe, we will learn another way of making smudge bundles.

Base: lavender, rosemary, sage, cedar, and rose petals

Other Materials Required

- 100 percent cotton thread or hemp string

- Scissors

Procedure

- Harvest your herbs.

- Cut them to the desired height.

- Begin bundling up the herbs. I prefer you start with the woodier herbs than the softer herbs. So, start with rosemary, then sage around it, then move on to the softer ones.

- Wrap the bundles once satisfied with their thickness. Wrap as tightly as possible from the roots upwards to the leaves (you can leave the leaves unwrapped).

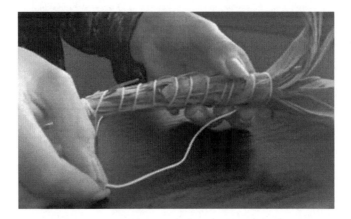

- Finally, hang the bundles to dry, and you will be done!

Incense Recipe 20

In this recipe, we will learn how to make smokeless incense. This is for you if you live in a small space or have issues with smoke, especially from incense made with charcoal.

Base: charcoal tablet

Liquid: Water

Bonding Agent: Rose essential oil

Other Materials Required

- Mortar and pestle

- Containers

- Spoon

Procedure

- Put the charcoal tablet in your mortar, then grind it till it turns to a fine powder.

- Add water to the charcoal. A few drops at a time will do.

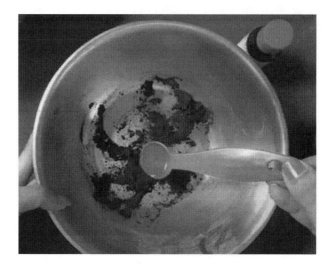

- Knead the charcoal well. Be careful not to add too much water as you make the dough. However, in case this happens, grind another charcoal disk, then use the powder.

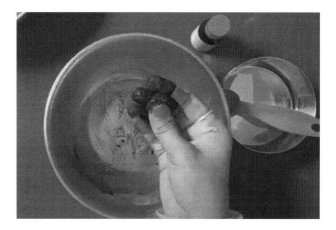

- Add some drops of rose essential oil to the dough. After a few drops, continue kneading well till you are satisfied that the oil has reached every part.

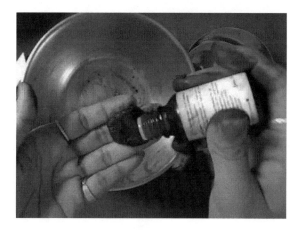

- Finally, shape the dough as a cone, then let it dry.

Incense Recipe 21

In this recipe, we will learn how to make incense without resins.

Base: bay leaves, cloves, cinnamon, and basil

Other Materials Required

- Salad bowl

- Wine glass or any type of container

- Wooden spoons or any other types of measuring spoons

- Salt

- Plastic ice cream dipper spoon

- Glue

- Paper

- Sieve

Procedure

- Pour salt into the wine glass or any container you will be using. The amount to use depends on the amount of incense you need.

- Put some bay leaves in the bowl, then grind it till it turns to a fine powder.

- Add clove to the bowl, then grind it. If you will use clove powder, add a half teaspoon.

- Take cinnamon, add it to the bowl, then grind. If you will be using powder, add half of a teaspoon.

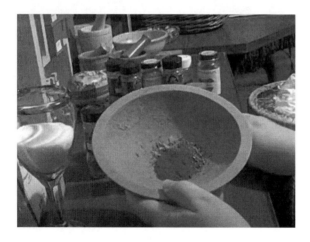

- Once the base materials are added to the bowl, mix them using a spoon.

- If you notice that some of the particles have not yet been grounded as required, grind them further using the bottom of a spice container, spice grinder, or a wooden spoon.

- Take a cylindrical object and wrap a piece of paper around it. What we want is to create a tube-like shape

- Deep the shaped paper in salt, then fill it with the incense. To avoid spilling, use a small sieve.

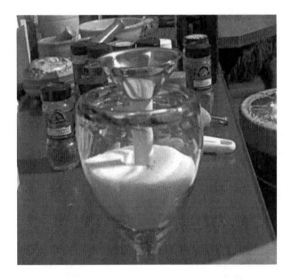

- Finally, light up your incense!

Incense Recipe 22

In this recipe, we will learn how to make black charcoal incense for hex breaking.

Base: Sage, rosemary, and ground cloves

Other Materials Required

- Charcoal disks or activated charcoal

- Dead sea salt

- Mortar and pestle

- Spoon

Procedure

- Use your mortar and pestle to grind the charcoal disks. If you are using activated charcoal, there will be no need to grind it because it comes mostly in powder form.

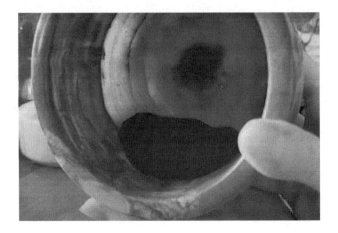

- Add some sage and rosemary to the charcoal, then grind them until they become a fine powder.

- Add cloves to the ground mixture, then continue grinding.

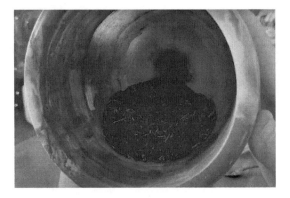

- Slowly pour the salt into the bowl. As you pour, stir it with a spoon.

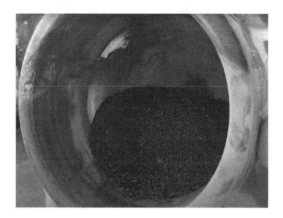

- Finally, pour some incense into an incense burner, and you are done!

Incense Recipe 23

In this recipe, we will learn how to make smudge incense for spiritual protection. This incense recipe has five essential herbs to help remove arguments, fights, evil eyes, and negative energy.

Base: cloves, hyssop, star anise, peppermint, ginger, nettle, and rosemary

Liquid: Water

Bonding Agent: Makko powder or what is known as tabu no ki powder

Other Materials Required

- String

- Scissors

Procedure

- Go to the garden or purchase fresh herbs from the list we have given above.

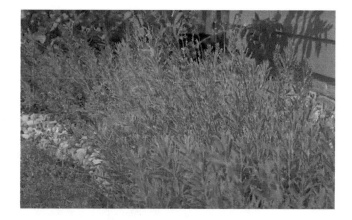

- Bundle sections of herbs from each herb category.

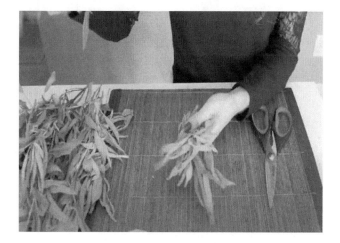

- Take some string and use it to tightly wrap the bundles created.

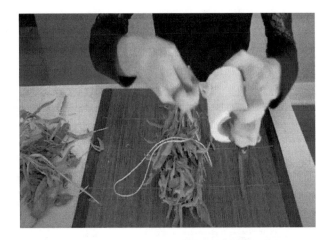

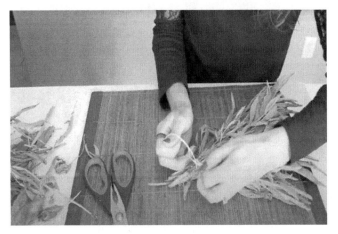

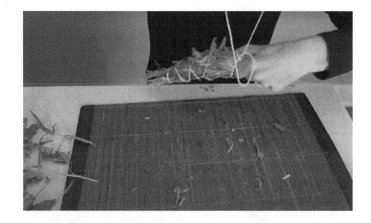

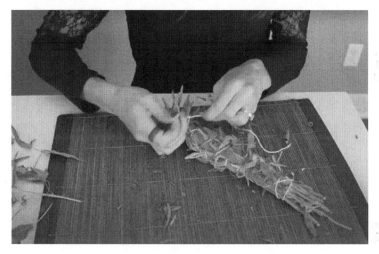

Once you get the number of bundles you need, light them as you require and enjoy!

Incense Recipe 24

In this recipe, we will learn how to make a love spell incense using essential oils.

Base: rose, apple, avocado leaves, basil, cinnamon, clove, rosemary, lavender, lemon balm, and vanilla fragrance oils

Bonding Agent: DPG essential oil

Other Materials Required

- Measuring scales

- Containers

- Spoon

- Unscented incense sticks

- Trays

- Plastic paper

- Paper towel

Procedure

- Measure 2 ounces of DPG essential oil and pour it into a container.

- Measure 1 ounce of fragrance oil and pour it into a container.

- Add the DPG oil to the love spell fragrance oil, then mix well with a spoon.

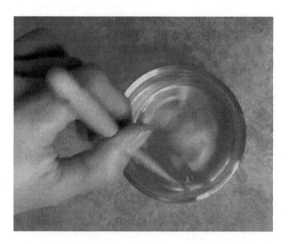

- Pour the fragrance oil into the tray.

- Spread the unscented incense sticks in a tray. The tray should be big enough to hold the sticks. In addition, roll the sticks to ensure that the fragrance touches all the incense stick corners.

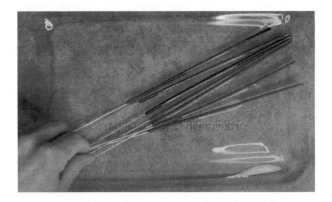

- Let the sticks soak for at least 24 hours. Before you begin the 24-hour countdown, cover the tray with plastic paper.

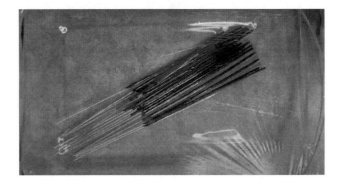

- After the 24-hour time elapses, spread them on a paper towel to dry. Dry them for at least 3 days, and after that, they will be ready for use!

Incense Recipe 25

In this recipe, we will learn how to make incense that helps cleanse your space while removing any type of negativity or stress.

Base: black sage, cedar, neem stems, and palo santo

Liquid: rose water

Bonding Agent: Makko powder or what is known as tabu no ki powder and ghee

Other Materials Required

- Containers

- Charcoal

- Mortar and pestle

- Standard cooking pan

- Lighter

Procedure

- Grind all the bases we have mentioned above then place them aside in a container or dish. You can grind one after the other or all at once – the aim is to ensure that the powder produced is as fine as possible.

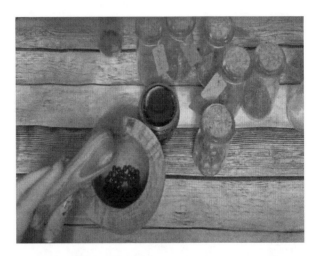

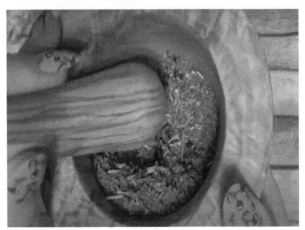

- Take a pan and put a piece of charcoal on it, then light it. Look at the image below:

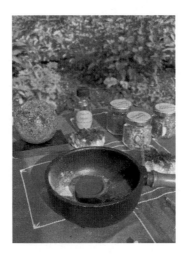

- Let the charcoal burn, then pinch by pinch, add the ground incense and enjoy!

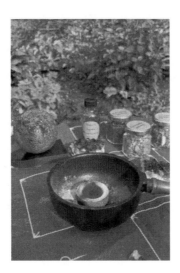

Incense Recipe 26

In this recipe, we will learn how to make incense that will help reduce pain and alleviate certain chronic illnesses and inflammation. In simple terms, this incense has powerful healing compounds.

Base: lavender, dandelion, peppermint, turmeric, aloe vera, ginger, rosemary, sage, chamomile, and ginkgo biloba

Liquid: Water

Bonding Agent: Makko powder

Other Materials Required

- Container

- Spoon

- Dropper

- Conical-shaped metal tips

- Twist tie

- Fan

- Heat-resistant container

- Sand

Procedure

- Grind all your bases separately, then put them aside in different containers.

- Measure the bases you need, then put them in one big bowl or container.

- Mix the bases well.

- Add your bonding agent – makko powder, then mix well.

- Add water with a dropper to make a dough.

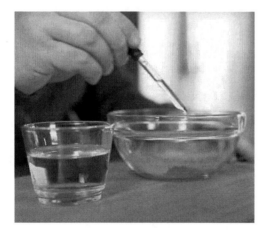

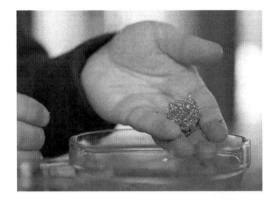

- Take conical-shaped metal tips (these are normally attached to icing bags for cake decorations), then fill them with the dough.

- To remove the molded cone, slip a twist tie into the tip.

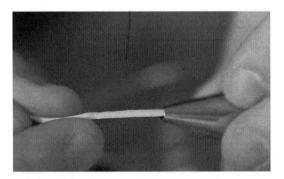

- Since the shaped incense has not yet dried up, lay it on a board line with wax paper.

- Lay the cones in the sun or a fan to dry. If you use the fan, set it on a 'low setting to dry. After 12 hours, lay them on their side. This will make it possible for them to dry all around.

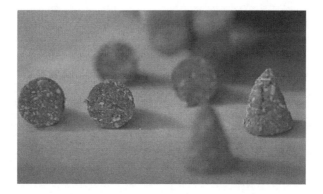

- Fill another container (the container should be heat-resistant) with sand, then lay your burning cone, and you are done!

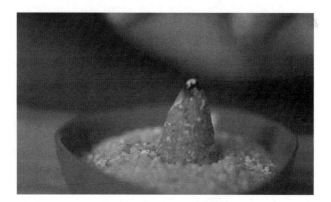

Incense Recipe 27

This recipe will teach us how to make incense to cure impotence and erectile dysfunction.

Base: tongkat ali, yohimbe bark, maca root, nan bao, sopalmito, ginkgo biluba extract, ginseng, and nutmeg

Liquid: Water and rose oil

Bonding Agent: Patchouli essential oil

Other Materials Required

- Containers

- Virgin olive oil

- Mortar and pestle

- Spoon

- Measuring scales or spoons

- Charcoal disk

- Cast iron cauldron

Procedure

The first thing to do is extract oil from ginkgo biloba leaves. To do this, follow the steps below;

- Fill a container or a glass jar with biloba leaves.

- Pour some virgin olive oil inside that same jar.

- Mix the biloba leaves properly with olive oil, then close the jar.

- Allow the leaves and the oil to cure for around six weeks. After six weeks, you will find some oil below the jar. This is the extract we need.

With the extract ready, let us go back to our bases.

- Grind tongkat ali, yohimbe bark, maca root, nan bao, sopalmito, ginseng, and nutmeg separately using a mortar and pestle, then put them aside.

- Grind makko, then put it aside.

- Measure and then mix the bases.

- Add a few drops of patchouli essential oil, then mix with a spoon.

- Add a few drops of rose oil, then mix with a spoon.

- Add half a teaspoon of honey, then mix with a spoon.

- Light a charcoal disk, then place it in the cast iron cauldron.

- Finally, pour some incense on top of the charcoal, and your incense is ready.

Incense Recipe 28

In this recipe, we will learn how to make incense to help with vaginal dryness. This incense has 13 herbs that help boost vaginal wetness when blended.

Base: Black cohosh, dong quai (also known as the female ginseng), linseed, fennel, fenugreek, sea buckthorn oil, red clover, aloe vera, manjistha, yashti, turmeric, madhu, shatavari

Liquid: Water

Bonding Agent: licorice root, dragon's blood resin, patchouli essential oil, and honey

Other Materials Required

- CO_2 extraction method tools

- Containers

- Measuring scales and/or spoons

- Charcoal

- Cast iron cauldron

- Lighter

- Incense tongs

Procedure

- Extract sea-buckthorn oil through the CO2 method.

This method involves grinding the sea-buckthorn berries and placing them in an extraction vessel. Next, put the Co2 gas under the vessel, which produces a high temperature.

Next, transmit the gas into an extraction vessel using a pump to break the berries down. Then, connect a pressure release valve to the pump to force the material into a different vessel. This material will be the oil we need.

- Once the sea buckthorn oil is extracted, put it aside.

- Grind all the other herbs separately using a mortar and pestle, then put them in different containers.

- Measure each herb, then put them in one big bowl or container. Mix well with a spoon.

- Grind your bonding agent, the licorice root, and dragon's blood, then add to the other herbs and mix well.

- Add the patchouli essential oil, then mix thoroughly. Add as you deem fit.

- Add honey and mix well. Add the amount as you deem fit.

- Add a few drops of patchouli essential oil, then mix with a spoon.

- Add a few drops of sea buckthorn extracted oil, then mix with a spoon.

- Light some charcoal, then place it in the cast iron cauldron.

- Finally, pour some incense on top of the charcoal, and your incense is ready!

Incense Recipe 29

In this recipe, we will learn how to make loose incense for magic.

Base: mandrake root, bay leaves, cinnamon roots, rosemary, yarrow, mugwort, belladonna, basil, lavender, rue, cloves

Liquid: lemon water

Other Materials Required

- Mortar and pestle

- Containers

- Spoon

- Soapstone incense burner

Procedure

- Grind all the bases one after the other using a mortar and pestle.

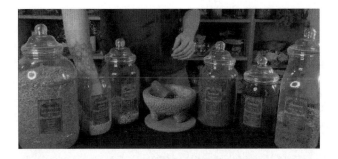

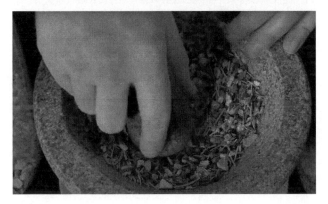

- Once the bases are grounded and mixed well using a spoon or by hand, add some lime water, then let it soak for 24 hours.

- Burn the mixed herbs using a soapstone oil burner. To do this, warm up the oil burner, then pour a small mixture on top.

- Since the burner is small, burn a small portion at a time.

Incense Recipe 30

This recipe will teach us how to make incense for better sleep and lucid dreaming.

Base: Mexican dream herb, mugwort, sun opener (heimia salicifolia), intellect tree (celastrus paniculatus), xhosa dream root (silene capensis), blue lotus (nymphaea caerulea), tian men dong, and the African dream bean

Liquid: Patchouli essential oil and rose water

Other Materials Required

- Charcoal tablets

- Knife

- Bowl

- Cast iron cauldron

- Lighter

- Incense tongs

- Containers

- Spoon

Procedure

- Grind each of the bases using a mortar and pestle, then put them in separate containers or jars.

- For easier grinding of woody herbs, especially if you purchase it in stick form, you might need to slice it with a craft knife or any other type of knife.

- Pour all the ingredients we have worked on so far into one bowl, then mix with a spoon.

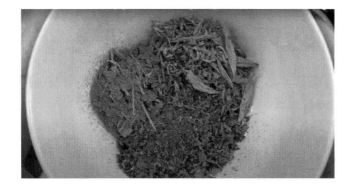

- Add a few drops of patchouli essential oil, then mix with a spoon.

- Add a few drops of rose oil, then mix.

- Add half a teaspoon of honey, and mix.

- Light some charcoal, then place it in the cast iron cauldron.

- Finally, pour some incense on top of the charcoal, and your incense is done!

Incense Recipe 31

In this recipe, we will learn how to make incense from essential oils. This incense will help you sleep better.

Base: Vetiver and lavender essential oils

Bonding Agent: DPG

Other Materials Required

- A two-and-a-half-gallon bucket or a tray big enough to house the whole unscented sticks

- Unscented incense sticks

- A bucket lid or plastic paper big enough to cover the tray

- Paper towel

Procedure

- Pour your fragrances into one jar, then mix with a spoon.

- Add DPG to the fragrances, then mix well with a spoon.

- Kindly note to use a 1:10 mixing ratio- this means 1 ounce of fragrance to every 10 ounces of DPG.

- Pour the mixture into the bucket or tray, then soak in the unscented incense sticks for at least 24 hours.

- Dry out the incense sticks on a paper towel for three days, and after that, burn them as you please!

Incense Recipe 32

In this recipe, we will learn how to make banishing incense using 20 herbs.

Base: tulsi, neem, chamomile, peppermint, rose, dill, oregano, parsley, sage, rosemary, cedar, lavender, bay leaves, juniper, frankincense, mugwort, St. John's wort, myrrh, and rue.

Other Materials Required

- Mortar and pestle

- Burning pot or dish

- Charcoal

Procedure

- Gather the bases we have listed above as bases.

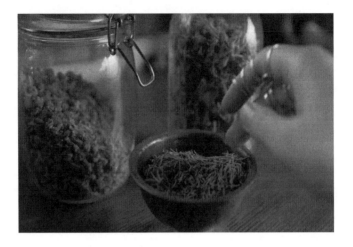

- Grind them in a mortar and pestle till they turn into a fine powder. You can grind one after the other or all at a go.

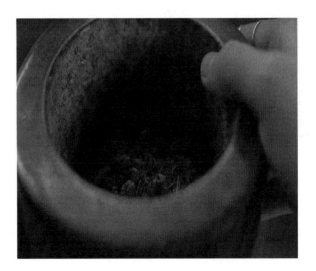

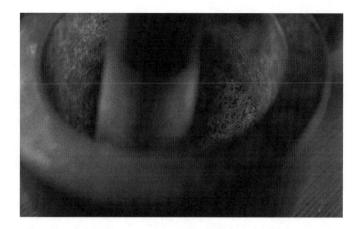

- Pour some charcoal into a burning pot or dish.

- Pour the ground mixture into a burning pot or dish.

- Finally, light the incense and enjoy.

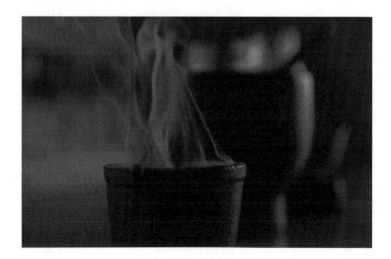

Incense Recipe 33

In this recipe, we will learn how to make incense that builds a fiery wall of protection from harmful energy or evil.

Base: Grains of paradise, cinnamon, ginger root, frankincense, sandalwood, red pepper, bay leaves, myrrh, rue, angelica root, and cayenne pepper

Bonding Agent: Dragon's blood, myrrh oil, olive oil, and frankincense oil

Other Materials Required

- Mortar and pestle or coffee grinder

- Containers or Petri dishes

- Spoon

Procedure

- Use mortar and pestle to grind each of the bases we have listed above. Use mortar and pestle. You can also use a coffee grinder.

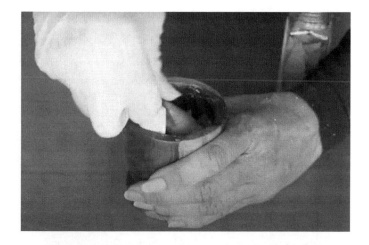

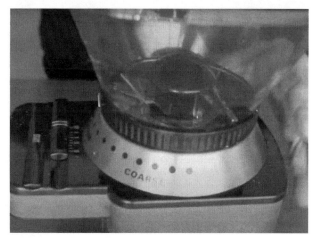

- After grinding them together, mix the bases together well, then put them in one container.

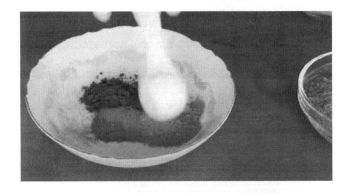

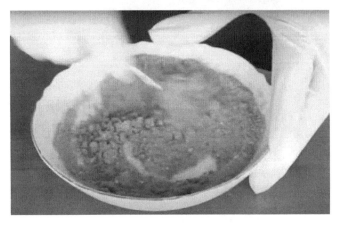

- Pour in a few drops of your bonding agents. I used dragon blood, myrrh, olive, and frankincense oil.

- Add water and work towards getting a dough.

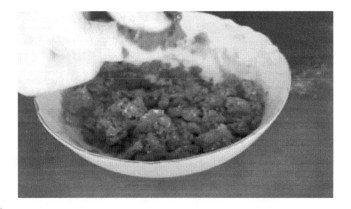

- Once a dough is made, mold them into cones.

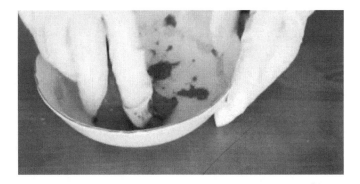

If you are having challenges molding the dough into a cone, you can get a piece of paper, roll it to a point then insert the dough in it. Look at the images below:

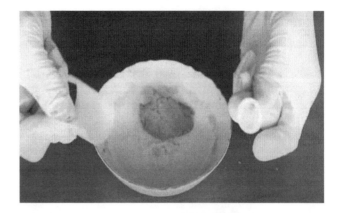

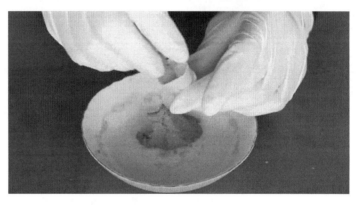

- Unroll the paper and assess the shape of the cone created.

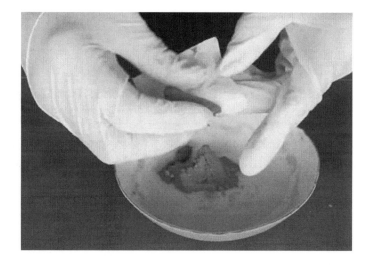

- Repeat the process till you get the number of cones you need.

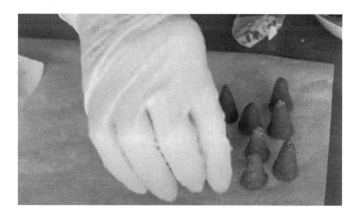

- Finally, let the cones dry for at least 24 hours, then use them when you please.

Incense Recipe 34

In this recipe, we will learn how to make incense from black salt. This incense will help protect you from hexes, wards, and spells.

Base: Rue, rosemary, mugwort, frankincense, and sage

Other Materials Required

- Organic activated black salt

- Gourmet black salt

- Lighter

- Charcoal briquette

- Incense burner

- Mortar and pestle

Procedure

- Light your charcoal briquette, then place it on an incense burner. Hold it using some incense tongs as you light the briquette.

- First, burn some mugwort, then let it burn a bit.

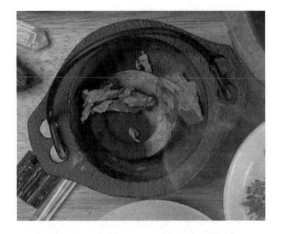

- Add some rue and let it burn.

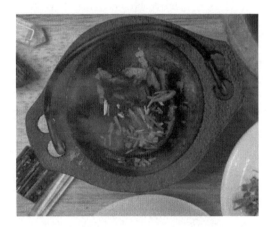

- Next, add rosemary, frankincense, and sage, respectively.

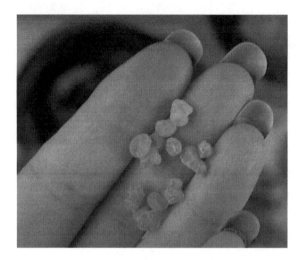

- As you can see from the above image, frankincense comes in chunks. You can drop it in the burner as it is, but you can also grind it using a mortar and pestle.

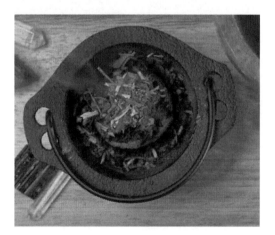

- Allow the whole mixture to burn completely; this will last for two hours or so. Below is the result;

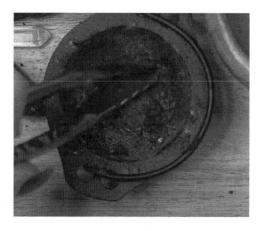

- Let the black powder cool down, then empty it all in a mortar.

- Grind the black powder further till it becomes finer.

- Add salt to the mortar, then continue grinding.

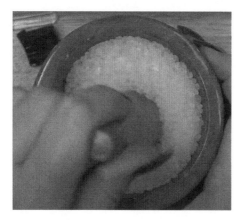

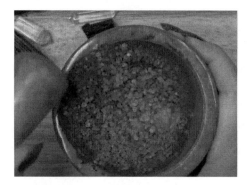

- If you want the salt darker, grind a charcoal briquette, then add it to the mixture.

- Finally, take the mixture back to the incense burner, then burn the desired amount as you want.

Incense Recipe 35

In this recipe, we will learn how to make incense from three common bases – lavender, rosemary, and white sage.

Base: White sage, rosemary, and lavender

Liquid: Water

Bonding Agent: Makko powder

Other Materials Required

- Rubber gloves

- Stirring sticks or popsicle sticks

- Syringe for measurements

- Cauldron

- Water

- Containers

- Spoon

Procedure

- Grind the three bases separately using a mortar and pestle.

- Pour the ground herbs into a cauldron. You can do an equal measure of each herb powder.

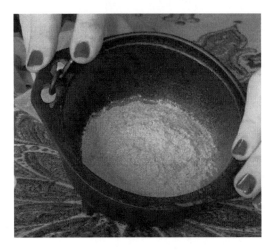

- Mix the herbs using a spoon.

- Grind your bonding agent, makko, add it to the herb mixture, then mix well with a spoon or the sticks.

- Use the syringe to measure some water, then pour it on the herb mixture.

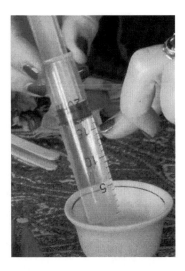

- Continue adding water sparingly till the mixture becomes chunky.

- Put on your gloves, then knead further. Add more water if you feel the dough is not perfect. Remember always to add it sparingly because we do not want the dough sticky.

- Take a chunk of the dough, then make shapes such as cones.

- Once the cones are done, let them dry for at least 4 days, but I recommend allowing them dry for a week or two.

- After they dry up, you can freely use them!

Incense Recipe 36

In this recipe, we will learn how to make third-eye incense. This incense will boost your psychic power, vision, and dream work. We will make this incense from herbal essential oils.

Base: Blue lotus, mugwort, angelica, wood betony, yarrow, sage, bay leaves, and jasmine flowers essential oils.

Other Materials Required

- Containers

- Cheesecloth lined trainer

- Unscented incense sticks

- Foil

- Flash tray with raised sides

- Gloves

Procedure

- Since we are handling essential oils, the first step is to measure equal quantities of the essential oils we have listed as the bases and then mix them in one main container.

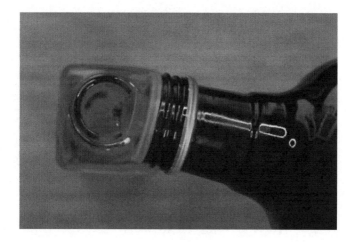

- Cover the tray with the foil paper.

- Lay the unscented incense sticks on the tray covered with foil paper.

- Pour the mixture of essential oils on the unscented incense sticks.

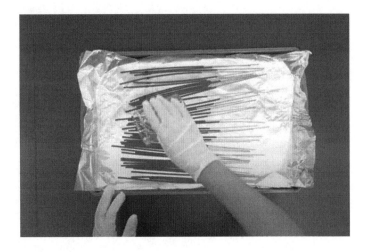

- Using your hands carefully, but for over 5 minutes, roll the incense sticks until the essential oils touch every part of them.

- Let the incense sticks cure for at least 30 minutes.

- Wrap the incense sticks with the foil paper, then let them cure further for over 4 hours.

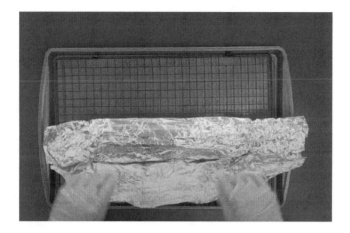

- Unwrap the incense sticks, then let them air dry for a week.

- If the sticks are still damp even after 24 hours, lay them on a paper towel. Let them dry up.

- Once dry, use them as you please!

Incense Recipe 37

In this recipe, we will learn how to make herbal incense for general yoga or meditation.

Base: Shatavari, shilajit, hartaki, amlaki, pipul, tulsi, brahmi, and aswagandha essential oils

Bonding Agent: DPG oil

Other Materials Required

- Olive dish

- Spoons

- Containers

- Large bowl

- Unscented incense sticks

- Paper towel

- Measuring spoons and scales s

Procedure

- Measure 1 pound from every essential oil. Be keen to measure only 1 ounce because this will determine the result.

- Pour your fragrances into one jar, then mix with a spoon.

- Use a measuring spoon or a pipette to measure 10 ounces of DPG.

- Add DPG to the fragrances, then mix well with a spoon.

- Pour the mixture into the tray or olive dish, then soak in the unscented incense sticks for at least 24 hours.

- Dry out the incense sticks on a paper towel for three days, and after that, burn them as you please!

Incense Recipe 38

In this recipe, we will learn how to make herbal incense that can be used during ayurveda yoga (this is a type of yoga that uses techniques such as chanting and yoga postures to treat mental and physical illnesses)

Base: Shatavari, shilajit, haritaki, amlaki, pipul, tulsi, brahmi, and aswagandha.

Color: Brown

Bonding Agent: licorice root, patchouli essential oil, and rose oil

Other Materials Required

- Mortar and pestle

- Spoon

- Lighter

- Knife

- Bowl

- Charcoal

- Cast iron cauldron

- Lighter

- Incense tongs

Procedure

- Put one base after another in a mortar and pestle, then grind them all.

- After you are done grinding the herbs above, put them aside in another container.

- Grind licorice root, our bonding agent then put it in a separate container.

- Pour all the ingredients we have worked on so far into one bowl, then mix with a spoon.

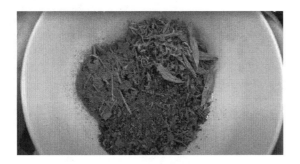

- Add a few drops of patchouli essential oil, then mix with a spoon.

- Add a few drops of rose oil, then mix.

- Light some charcoal, then place it in the cast iron cauldron.

- Finally, pour some incense on top of the charcoal, and you will be done!

Incense Recipe 39

In this recipe, we will learn how to make herbal incense that can be used during yoga to increase vitality and physical energy. Specifically, it will help boost, ojas, vital energy, and soma.

Base: makhana, lotus stem, kapikacchu, dioscorea, ginseng, shilajit vidari, bala, shatavari, amalaka, and ashwagandha

Bonding Agent: honey

Other Materials Required

- Charcoal tablets

- Knife

- Bowl

- Cast iron cauldron

- Lighter

- Incense tongs

- Containers

- Spoon

Procedure

- Grind each of the bases using a mortar and pestle, then put them in separate containers or jars.

- For easier grinding of woody herbs, especially if you purchase it in stick form, you might need to slice it with a craft knife or any other type of knife.

- Pour all the ingredients we have worked on so far into one bowl, then mix with a spoon.

- Add a few drops of honey, then mix with a spoon.

- Light some charcoal, then place it in a cast iron cauldron.

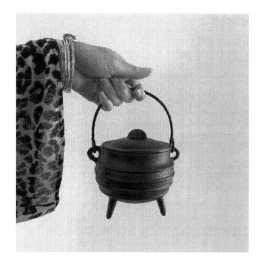

- Finally, pour some incense on top of the charcoal, and your incense is done!

Incense Recipe 40

In this recipe, we will learn how to make herbal incense that can be used during yoga to cleanse your body, the whole nervous system in particular.

Base: manduka parni, brahmi, gotu kola, barberry, gentian, guduchi, turmeric, and aloe gel

Bonding Agent: makko powder and honey

Other Materials Required

- Containers

- Mortar and pestle

- Incense burner

- Charcoal disks

- Tongs

- Foil paper

- Candle

- Sieve

- Candle container

- Foil paper

Procedure

- Grind the bases using a mortar and pestle, then place them in containers. You can grind one after the other if you have a big grinder or mortar and pestle.

- Grind the makko powder, then pour it into the container with the powder bases.

- Stir everything well with a spoon.

- Add honey.

- Stir everything together nicely.

- Depending on how consistent you want the mixture to be, add more honey as you continue the stirring but do not make the mixture too sticky.

- Set up your tea light incense warmer.

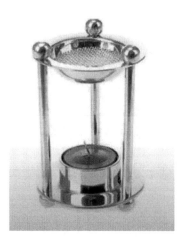

- This is a candle holder with a sieve on top. So, put a candle inside and the incense on top of the sieve. Before you pour the incense into the sieve, line it with foil paper.

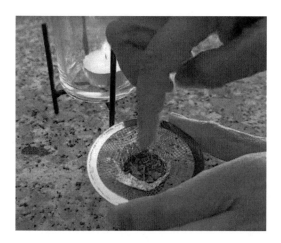

- And your incense is ready!

Incense Recipe 41

In this recipe, we will learn how to make herbal incense that will help stimulate your senses and mind and improve your perception. This recipe will also help remove mucus from the head and boost cerebral circulation.

Base: elecampe, sage, ephedra, bayberry, long pepper or long pepper, basil, tulsi, and calamus or vacha

Liquid: Water

Bonding Agent: licorice root and lavender essential oil

Other materials required

- Mortar and Pestle

- Sieve

- Containers

- Wooden splits

- Kneading board

- Wax paper

Procedure

- Grind the 8 bases, then sieve them into different containers.

- Grind the licorice root and put it in a different container.

- Pour some drops of lavender essential oil on wax paper, then spread it.

- Pour all the bases into one big container or bowl, then mix thoroughly with a spoon.

- Add the licorice root powder to the bowl and mix once more.

- Place the dough on the wax paper, wrap it, then roll it with a kneading board.

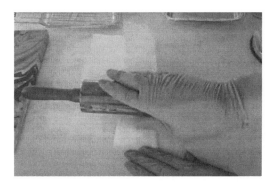

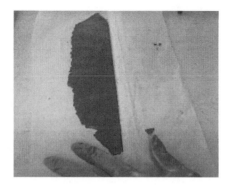

- Press a stick in the dough, then wrap it in the dough.

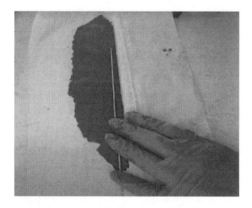

- Roll the sick on the board.

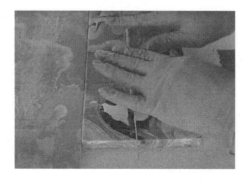

- Let the sticks dry, and you are done!

Incense Recipe 42

In this recipe, we will learn how to make herbal incense that will help strengthen your mind. This means that your concentration will be boosted.

Base: shilajit, lotus seeds, kapikacchu, bala, shatavari, harikati, ashagandha, manduka parni, brahmi,and shankha pushpi

Liquid: Rose Water

Bonding Agent: licorice root

Other Materials Required

- Trays

- Mortar and pestle

- Containers

- Standard drinking straws

- Slim chopsticks

Procedure

- Dry all your herbs if you are harvesting or purchasing them fresh.

- Dry the base herbs one after another, then mix them together nicely.

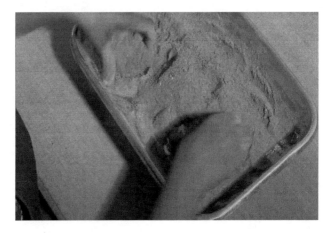

- Grind the bonding agent, licorice root using your mortar and pestle.

- Add the bonding agent to the base mixture.

- Add some water sparingly to the mixture, then make a dough by mixing and then kneading it.

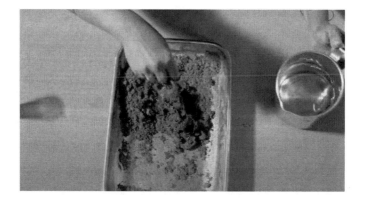

- Once you get a fairly sticky dough, you can roll it into sticks or push them through drinking straws to make incense sticks. If you use straws, use sticks as long as chopsticks to push the incense sticks out.

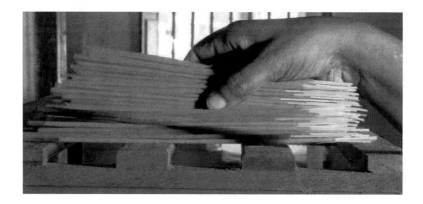

- You can also make cones from the same mixture.

- Once done making your incense sticks and cones, let them dry for at least a week or so, and they will be ready for use!

Incense Recipe 43

In this recipe, we will learn how to make herbal incense that will help slow down your mind during meditation. In addition, this incense will help reduce any agitated nerves and significantly reduce anxiety.

Base: lady's slipper, kava kava, passion flower, sandalwood, nutmeg, ashwagandha, valerian, and the jatamansi

Liquid: Water

Bonding Agent: licorice root

Other Materials Required

- Sieve

- Grinder or mortar and spice

- Spoon

- Containers

Procedure

- Get your dry lady's slipper, kava kava, passion flower, sandalwood, nutmeg, ashwagandha, valerian, and the jatamansi, then grind them together.

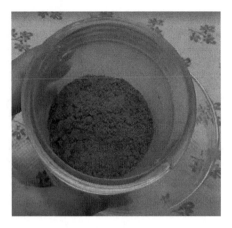

- Sieve the ground bases into a bigger container.

- Grind licorice root either using a mortar and pestle or using an electric herb grinder

- Add the licorice powder, then mix well.

- Add water to the mixture, then mix till it turns into a dough, but the dough should not be sticky

- Take a piece of plastic paper, then shape it into a cone shape. To keep the shape together, seal it with a piece of tape.

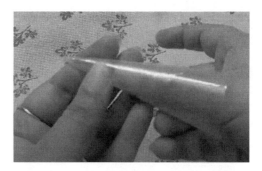

- Fill the cone with the mixture.

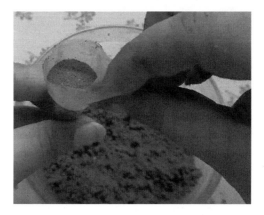

- After pressing the mixture down, slide it out of the plastic shaped-cone.

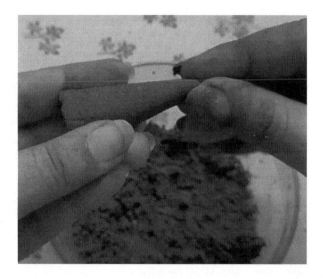

- Let the cones dry for three days, and you are done!

Incense Recipe 44

In this recipe, we will learn how to make herbal incense for athletes! This incense will help boost your athletic performance in general. Specifically, this incense will help increase stamina, reduce inflammation as you work out, shorten the recovery time, and improve reaction times and reflexes!

You can use these ingredients to make cones, sticks, or smudge bundles. In this project, we will make smudge bundles.

Base: ginseng, cat's claw, maca, guarana, turmeric, boswllia serrata, and eleuthero root

Liquid: Water

Bonding Agent: licorice root

Other Materials Required

- Cotton thread

Procedure

- Harvest fresh ginseng, cat's claw, maca, guarana, turmeric, Boswellia serrata, and eleuthero root.

- Take a bunch from each type of flower, bundle them together, then wrap them with cotton threads.

- Kindly note that the thread should be wrapped tightly, and it should be passed in both directions.

- Hang them to dry in a well-ventilated place that is away from direct sunlight.

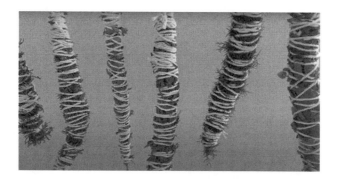

- Once dry, which will take around two weeks, it is ready to burn!

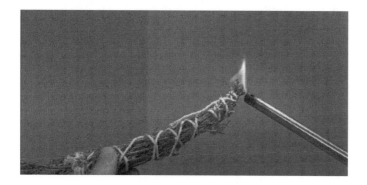

Incense Recipe 45

In this recipe, we will learn how to make herbal incense for spiritual enlightenment. If you are having interpersonal connection issues, this incense is for you!

Please note that the base list is long, but you are free to choose what you prefer.

Base: basil, aloe vera, sage, mint, vetiver, lavender, jasmine, thyme, rosemary, peacy lily, Chinese money plant, jade plant, calatheas, and eucalyptus.

Other Materials Required

- Bamboo tree

- Organic activated black salt

- Gourmet black salt

- Lighter

- Charcoal briquette

- Incense burner

- Mortar and pestle

Procedure

- Light your charcoal briquette, then place it on an incense burner. Hold it using some incense tongs as you light the briquette.

- First, burn some peacy lily, then let it burn a bit.

- Add one base after the other. Only add another base if the other one starts burning.

- Allow the whole mixture to burn completely.

- Burning may take longer than the standard two hours because our list of bases is longer.

- Below is the result;

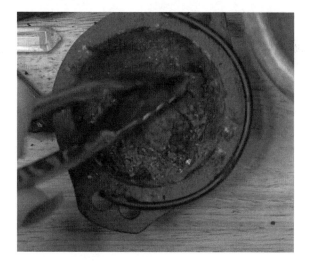

- Let the black powder cool down, then empty it all in a mortar.

- Grind the black powder further.

- Add salt to the mortar, then continue grinding.

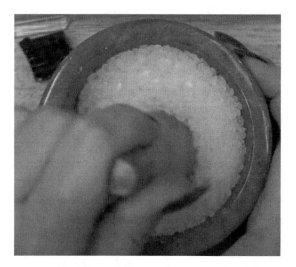

- Finally, take the mixture back to the incense burner, then burn the desired amount as you want.

Incense Recipe 46

In this recipe, we will learn how to make Tibetan herbal incense

Please note that the base list is long, but you are free to choose what you prefer.

Base: Chinese caterpillar fungus, borneol, clove, red orpine, saffron, hibiscus, snow lotus, frankincense, amber, myrrh, cedar, pine, agar, and sandalwood

Liquid: Water

Bonding Agent: charcoal and makko powder

Other Materials Required

- Grinder or pestle and mortar

- Spoon

- Containers

- Water

- Incense blanks

- Matchbox

Procedure

- Grind all the bases one by one as you put them in separate containers.

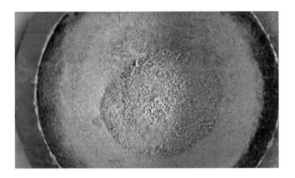

- After grinding all the bases, measure the amount you need from each, then transfer them into one bigger bowl.

- Pour makko powder into the big bowl, then mix thoroughly.

- Add some water. Be careful about adding the water because we do not want to make the mixture sticky.

- Knead the mixture as you continue adding water sparingly.

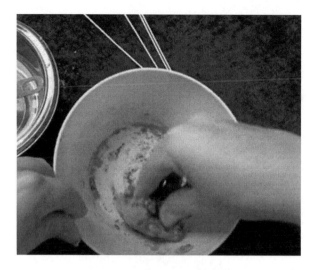

- Knead it till it gets a bread dough consistency.

- Once done, feel the dough. If it is sticky, add some makko powder, then continue kneading.

- Once the dough is ready, it is time to wrap it around the incense blanks. To do this, roll the dough into the size and length of the blanks.

- Once the rolled dough is big enough, take a blank and press it on the dough. Then roll the dough around the blank.

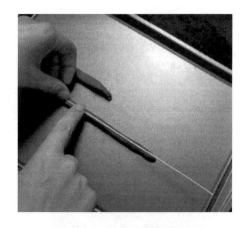

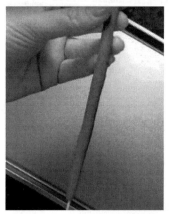

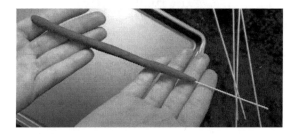

- You can also make cones from the dough too!

- Allow the incense to dry for at least three days and you are ready to use them!

Incense Recipe 47

In this recipe, we will learn how to make pine resin cones.

Base: Sandalwood dust, tragacanth, and pine

Liquid: Water

Other Materials Required

- Measuring spoons

- Containers

Procedure

- Measure 2 tablespoons of sandalwood dust and pour it into a container.

- Measure 1 tablespoon of pine resin and pour it into a container.

- Mix the two thoroughly.

- Store the mixture in a jar, then store it for a month.

- After 1 month of aging, pour the incense into a container.

- Add 1/8 of a full teaspoon of tragacanth gum powder to it.

- Add water to the mixture, then knead to make a dough.

- After the dough is made, cover it and let it cure for 24 hours.

- Shape the dough into cones.

- Let the shape dry for 24 hours, then use them.

Incense Recipe 48

In this recipe, we will learn how to make incense from royal resin oil. This incense can be made from raw resin, but in this recipe, we will learn how to extract the oil and use it to make sweet-smelling incense!

Base: Sweet myrrh, opal

Liquid: Water

Bonding Agent: Grapeseed oil

Other Materials Required

- Crockpot or two pots with lids

- Water

- Containers

- Jar or spray bottle

- Paper towel

- Plastic bag

- Spray bottle

Procedure

- Put opal chunks and the base in a jar. Work on a 1:5 ratio – if you put one ounce of the base, put 5 of the bonding agent.

- Fill the jar with grapeseed oil, then put it in the pot.

- Close the pot, then warm it for around 6 hours.

- Sieve the liquid into a clean jar or a spray bottle.

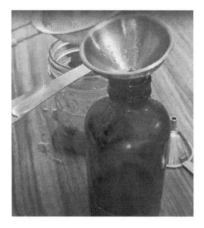

- Put unscented incense sticks in a paper bag and close it up for 24 hours to make them as dense as possible.

- After 24 hours, spray the bag with the extracted oil till the incense sticks look soaked.

- Close up the bag and let it cure for at least three days

- After three days, remove the incense sticks and spread them on a paper towel for at least 2 days.

- After they are dry, you are free to burn them!

Incense Recipe 49

In this recipe, we will learn how to make traditional Japanese incense.

Base: Cloves, spikenard valerian, costus root, ginger, vetivert, turmeric, borneol, myrrh, frankincense, patchouli leaves, cassia, cedarwood, aloeswood, sandalwood, and star anise.

Liquid: Water

Bonding Agent: Makko

Other Materials Required

- Mortar and pestle

- Containers

- Heat source

Procedure

- Grind the bases using a mortar and pestle to a powder form.

- Heat some water.

- Once in powder form, add warm or heated water.

- Knead the powder and water till it becomes dough.

- Form the dough into sticks or cones.

- Let the incense dry for at least a week at room temperature, and the incense will be ready!

Incense Recipe 50

In this recipe, we will learn how to make resin and gum incense.

Base: almond tree resin, Loban herb, black storax resin, copal resin, and dammar gun

Other Materials Required

- Incense burner

- Lighter

- Charcoal disks

- Bamboo charcoal

- Aloes gum

- Acacia gum

- Benzoin Sumatran

- Incense tongs

- Fireproof dish

Procedure

- Light the charcoal disk and place a heated bamboo charcoal then put it in an incense burner.

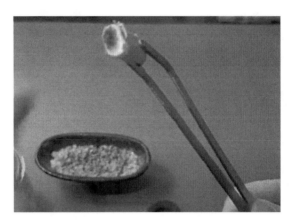

- You can also put some granulated salt in the dish and then place bamboo charcoal.

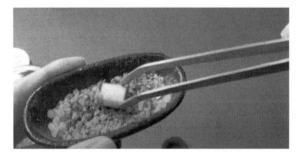

- Burn one resin after the other but wait for each to burn a bit before adding the next.

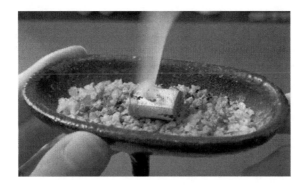

- Once done, and after all the resins and herbs are burned out, which is almost after two hours, you can decide to throw away the powder, or you can decide to re-use it.

- Re-using it is not challenging. All you have to do is, grind it further, place it in the dish then burn more resins.

Finally, once you make your incense, your tools will definitely be dirty. To clean them, read the next section.

Chapter 7: How to Clean Incense-Making Tools

Now, let us learn how to clean your tools;

- **Grinders**

If you were using electrical grinders, clean them by;

Materials required

- Water

- Paper towel

- A quarter cup of uncooked rice of any type

Procedure

- Measure and pour a quarter cup of rice into the grinder, then grind it for around one minute. Once done, you will notice some oil clinging to the rice and thin dust.

- Remove the rice flour, then wipe the grinder with a damp towel, and your grinder will be clean!

You can also do this;

- Take stale bread or dry bread, then put it in the grinder.

- Grind the bread for about 30 to 60 seconds, then remove what remains.

- Finally, clean the interior of the bowl and the grinder itself using a damp piece of cloth.

Cleaning the mortar and pestle is easier. All you have to do is;

- Lather a sponge with unscented soap, then use it to clean the mortar and pestle for about 5 minutes thoroughly.

- Heat some warm water, then rinse the mortar and pestle. Do this until all the soap residue is all gone.

- Dry the mortar and pestle using a dry piece of cloth, and your cleaning is done!

Note:

Use this last method to clean the tweezers and measuring spoons:

- **Incense burners**

To clean standard incense burners;

- Heat some water.

- Place the burner in a sink.

- Pour the warm water through the burner.

- If you do not want to run warm water through it, submerge the burner in the water.

- Let the water run through the burner for as long as possible (this means that the water you use should be in plenty). If you had submerged your burner in water, soak it for 10 to 15 minutes.

- Wipe down the burner using a sponge. The sponge will also help remove any residue left.

- Heat more water till it is warm, then do a final rinse.

- Finally, air-dry the burner, and you will be done!

You can also clean it through the following steps;

Materials required:

- Isopropyl alcohol

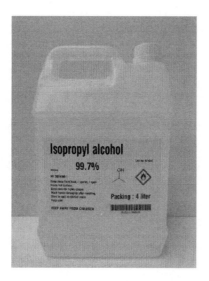

- Ziploc bag

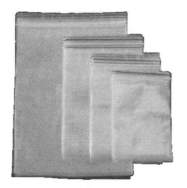

Procedure

- Choose a Ziploc bag that will fit your burner.

- Fill the bag with isopropyl alcohol, then put the burner in (you can also do this and vice versa).

- Shake the bag for around 10 minutes. Remove the burner from the bag; then air dry it.

- If you notice that there are parts that are not adequately clean, take a cotton swab and dip it in isopropyl alcohol, then work on the residue.

- If that does not work, dip a cotton ball in isopropyl alcohol, hold it with tweezers, and clean the hard-to-reach stained areas.

Conclusion

This book has proven that creating a relaxing atmosphere in your home or enhancing your spiritual practice without worrying about your respiratory system or illnesses that come with poorly-created incense is possible.

All you have to do is read and re-read this beginner's guide to making herbal incense and perfect your journey to making a natural, safe, and easy way to create beautiful scents for your home!

Good luck!

PS: I'd like your feedback. If you are happy with this book, please leave a review on Amazon.

Please leave a review for this book on Amazon by visiting the page below:

https://amzn.to/2VMR5qr

Made in the USA
Columbia, SC
13 April 2024

da09f4a2-53d2-4ae2-af34-63fabd22d526R01